FOCUS
ON
KIDS

Adolescent HIV Risk Prevention

University of Maryland
Department of Pediatrics

ETR Associates
Santa Cruz, California
1998

ETR Associates (Education, Training and Research) is a nonprofit organization committed to fostering the health, well-being and cultural diversity of individuals, families, schools and communities. The publishing program of ETR Associates provides books and materials that empower young people and adults with the skills to make positive health choices. We invite health professionals to learn more about our high-quality publishing, training and research programs by contacting us at P.O. Box 1830, Santa Cruz, CA 95061-1830, 1-800-321-4407.

Published by ETR Associates
P.O. Box 1830, Santa Cruz, CA 95061-1830.

Printed in the United States of America
10 9 8 7 6 5 4 3 2 1

ISBN 1-56071-591-X

Title No. R565

Contents

8 sessions
1.5 - 2.0 hrs

Acknowledgments

Over the last several years, we have had a wonderful and exciting time working with hundreds of youth, parents and organizations from Baltimore City to develop, implement, and evaluate the *Focus on Kids* HIV prevention curriculum. Everyone with whom we worked was committed to a common goal; to prevent our adolescents from becoming infected with HIV. It appears that all of our efforts have paid off; youth participating in the *Focus on Kids* programs are less likely to engage in HIV risk behaviors than youth who have not participated in this program. We are proud of this curriculum and hope that every one of the individuals and organizations with whom we have worked will share in this pride.

With the help of the Centers for Disease Control and Prevention, Division of Adolescent and School Health and ETR Associates, we are now able to make this curriculum available to other community workers throughout the United States. We have tried to make the curriculum sufficiently straightforward so that it can be understood by simply reading through it. We invite anyone to use any part of it (or all of it). All we ask is that you acknowledge us and that you occasionally give us feedback (whether good or bad) after you have used it.

We will also be available to offer training sessions in the curriculum for persons who deal professionally with early adolescents. Please contact Jennifer Galbraith at 410-706-4267 if you are interested in trainings.

When you use this curriculum, remember that you and the youth should be having fun. People learn more quickly if they enjoy what they are doing. The curriculum contains some factual information but really emphasizes decision making, communication and negotiation. We include a lot of practice examples. Like everything else in life, "practice makes perfect."

Focus on Kids could not have been made without the help of many individuals. We wish to thank all the youth and their parents who worked with us throughout the curriculum development and evaluation. We also want to thank the community interviewers and group leaders who worked with us and enabled us to evaluate the curriculum. We also must thank the staff of the many community recreation centers, Baltimore City Schools, the Housing Authority of Baltimore City and other agencies that helped us along the way.

The curriculum would not have been possible without the aid and funding of the National Institute of Mental Health, the National Institute of Child Health and Development, and the Agency for Health Care Policy and Research for supporting our efforts. The Child Health Foundation supported our efforts to turn the results of this work over to Baltimore City communities. Finally, we thank those at ETR Associates and the Centers for Disease Control and Prevention for aiding us in reaching a much greater audience of youth.

We dedicate this manual to the youth and families of Baltimore City.

The Focus on Kids Team

Introduction

What Is Focus on Kids?

Focus on Kids is a community-university linked research and intervention program. The goal of *Focus on Kids* is to reduce the risk of HIV infection among urban youth. The University of Maryland Department of Pediatrics works together with community members from recreation centers, housing developments, schools and government agencies to reach this goal.

The *Focus on Kids* program is built on a philosophy of education in which youth are provided both the knowledge and the skills they need to protect themselves from becoming infected with HIV.

What Makes Focus on Kids Different?

One unique aspect of the *Focus on Kids* program is that it has been conducted exclusively in recreation centers as opposed to schools or clinics. The purpose of this community basis for the program is to reach higher-risk youth who are already truant from school or have high absenteeism rates and those youth who do not go to clinics or are not connected with health care professionals. It also allows the behavior change prevention program to be closer to where youth will be making decisions about high-risk activities—in their neighborhoods and social networks.

Another unique aspect of *Focus on Kids* is its emphasis on community involvement. The community has been involved in the project on many different levels. Initially, several recreation club directors were hired as consultants to help the research team better understand the youth and the best way to reach them. A community advisory board was also formed. The board has been an invaluable component and has aided in survey and curriculum development, as well as the overall design of the project.

Focus on Kids has also tried to use community members in as many roles as possible—as interviewers, group leaders and research assistants. Through our work with the community, we were able to gain insight into the needs and perceptions of urban youth and their parents.

Focus on Kids is also unique in it's use of "natural friendship groups." As each young person enrolled in the original *Focus on Kids* program, he or she was asked to invite 3 to 9 same-gender friends to join the program, thus forming natural friendship groups. In this way, the young people were able to reinforce each other's positive, healthy decisions.

Although *Focus on Kids'* primary goal was to reduce HIV infection, the team was aware that there are many things that lead to risk behaviors among youth, and that it therefore was important to make the curriculum holistic and comprehensive. It became obvious from talking with parents, youth and community leaders who work with youth that the curriculum would need to be broad and cover many topics, including decision making, values clarification, communication, and knowledge about risk behaviors associated with HIV infection, other STD, teen pregnancy, violence, drug use and drug selling.

Program History

Focus on Kids began with a team of researchers consisting of pediatricians, psychologists, health educators and anthropologists. Through these multiple disciplines, the *Focus on Kids* team was able to approach the numerous challenges which face urban youth in the 1990s from epidemiological, individual and community perspectives. From these perspectives, the team developed a curriculum based on social cognitive theory. Ethnographic and survey research, as well as strong community input, ensured that the intervention was developmentally and culturally grounded.

During the spring of 1993, *Focus on Kids* was ready to try the curriculum with a large number of youth to determine if it would actually decrease risk behaviors for HIV infection. For this study, 383 youth, ages 9–15, from 9 recreation centers in urban, low-income neighborhoods of Baltimore were enrolled. All youth were African American.

Youth were given information on the project and a permission slip for their parents to sign to be enrolled. If youth were interested in joining the project, they were asked to invite up to 9 of their same-sex friends to join the program with them.

Altogether there were 76 of these "friendship groups." The hope was that by working with groups of friends, youth would be more likely to want to come to the group meetings. The team also anticipated that youth would encourage each other to change behavior, and that peer pressure would work to change behavior in a positive direction.

The friendship groups were selected at random to receive either the *Focus on Kids* curriculum or a strictly factual curriculum. At the completion of the intervention, each peer group had the option of either working one-on-one as peer educators with community members, or of working together as a group to produce a product that would deliver a message about HIV prevention to a particular population. The youth could choose the content of the message, the target audience, and the medium through which the message would be delivered. Youth-driven projects included a video, the painting of posters, and the production of a play.

Evaluation and Results

The *Focus on Kids* program was evaluated to determine if it had reached its goal of decreasing risk behaviors among the participants. Youth were given questionnaires that surveyed their knowledge, attitudes and risk behaviors around HIV before the program began, and then again at 6, 12, 18 and 24 months after the program.

Before the program, condom-use rates did not differ significantly between the group receiving the *Focus on Kids* curriculum and the group receiving the factual curriculum.

At 6 months post-intervention, condom–use rates were significantly higher among youth who participated in the *Focus on Kids* curriculum (85%) than they were among control youth (61%) ($p<0.05$). Condom–use intention, measured by a 5-point Likert-type scale, was also increased among *Focus on Kids* youth at 6 months (2.84 vs. 3.34, $p<0.01$). Some perceptions about condom use were also positively affected at 6 months.

Future Goals

Although the *Focus on Kids* curriculum has been proven successful at reducing risk factors among adolescents, to be truly successful many more youth need to be reached. Thanks to the Centers for Disease Control and Prevention's Research to Classroom Project this goal can now be achieved.

In addition, 2 spin-off programs from *Focus on Kids* have been started: Pilot Light trains recreation club directors in the *Focus on Kids* curriculum so that it may be delivered on a more continuous basis, and Project ImPACT works with parents and youth together to increase communication and parents' monitoring skills.

Getting Started

How many youth should be in a group?

The curriculum was designed for and works best with groups of 6 to 10 youth.

How do I form a group of youth?

Focus on Kids used "natural friendship groups" or youth who already spent time together. The hope is that if youth are friends, they can help support each other with the skills they are being taught. Working with groups of friends also may make youth more likely to come to the group meetings. Recreation clubs (e.g., drama club), arts and crafts, dance groups, church clubs, scouting groups or sports teams might be a way to find friendship groups. You also could approach several youth and suggest they get some of their friends together to form a group.

Can I run a group by myself?

The original program was done with 2 group leaders, and this seems to work best. By co-facilitating, one group leader is free to deal with a youth who is having behavioral problems while the other can continue with the rest of the group. Co-facilitators also can model good communication and negotiation skills for youth.

Having 2 group leaders incorporates different styles and personalities, which can enable more youth to be reached. Group leaders might have different strengths (e.g., one might be an older professional with lots of experience, and the other be closer to the age of the group members). Although it is possible to do *Focus on Kids* with a single group leader, we strongly recommend co-facilitating.

How often should I run the groups?

The curriculum was designed for 1 session per week; however, you can be flexible with scheduling. You might want to meet twice a week instead. It is important to meet at a regular time each week so youth know when the group meeting is.

What if youth don't come back?

There are various ways to help ensure youth enjoy the program and keep coming back.

- First, make the group meetings fun; keep them upbeat and active.

- You may also want to introduce some incentives such as snacks, certificates or small gifts. (See Resource Section for Tips on Soliciting Donations.)

- You can agree to place 50¢ or $1 in a group "bank account" every time youth come. The money can be used for a group outing of the youths' choice at the end of the program.

- Finally, call and remind youth about the program, do home visits, send out postcards and have youth remind each other.

What about parents?

Parents need to be told what the program is about and should sign a parent permission slip. (An outline for a Parent Information Session and a Sample Parent Permission Slip are provided in the Resource Section.) Ensuring that parents have bought into the program is important. An information session for parents can explain what the program is about and allow parents to experience some of the activities used in the curriculum.

What age should the youth be?

The program was designed for and has been shown to work with youth 9 to 15 years of age. Because of the large developmental gap between a 9 year old and a 15 year old, it's important to have no more than a 3-year age difference between members in a group (i.e., 9–12, 11–14, or 12–15). Many of the activities in the curriculum are adapted for specific age groups. The symbol [YOUNGER YOUTH] indicates activities that are more appropriate for youth in the 9- to 12-year-old age range; the symbol [OLDER YOUTH] indicates activities that have been adapted for the 12- to 15-year-old age range.

How do I make this program relevant for youth in my community?

As mentioned previously, the *Focus on Kids* curriculum is based on social cognitive theory, and ethnographic and survey research was conducted to ensure that the intervention was developmentally and culturally grounded. The target audience for *Focus on Kids* was urban youth, ages 9–15, from predominantly low-income areas, all of whom were African American. Although this was the audience that *Focus on Kids* was designed for, the curriculum is still relevant for many other adolescent groups; however, it may be necessary to make minor adaptations to best suit the needs of your targeted community.

One strategy that might help when adapting the curriculum is to have an advisory board made up of community leaders (e.g., teachers, rec club directors, church leaders), parent and youth from your community. Share the curriculum with the advisory board and listen to their recommendations on what might need to be altered. Another strategy is to conduct a few focus group meetings with groups of 8–10 parents or youth where you ask what their concerns are and what they feel youth need to learn to protect themselves. A final strategy is to get survey information, if it is available, to determine what risk behaviors are most common among the youth with whom you will be working.

There is limited information about alcohol use in the *Focus on Kids* curriculum because the data showed that this risk behavior was not prevalent among the original target population. Drug selling, however, was a concern heard frequently from parents and youth, so the curriculum places a greater emphasis on preventing drug selling. Minor changes to the curriculum can help ensure you are best addressing the needs of your youth.

What about youth who want to join the group later?

After the second or third session it is difficult for youth to join and get all the information needed. It is therefore best to close the group at this time and have youth wait until you are able to start a new group.

Should I have boys and girls in the same group?

The curriculum was designed for single sex groups; however, it is a good idea to combine girls' and boys' groups occasionally so participants can hear how the other gender thinks and can practice roleplaying in mixed-gender groups.

One possibility for bringing boys and girls together is an all-day retreat (see below).

How does the all-day retreat work?

In the original *Focus on Kids* program, an all-day retreat was offered during Session 6 as an incentive for youth who had attended 3 or more sessions. Youth were taken to a camp outside the city where they participated in the educational activities in Session 6, as well as recreational activities.

The retreat is an ideal time to bring a speaker in to talk to all of the groups at one time. Possible speakers include a person living with HIV or someone from the community sharing his or her life experiences. Check with your local health department, family planning agencies or HIV organizations to see if they have a speakers bureau.

The retreat also offers an opportunity for groups of boys and girls to come together to understand the others' perceptions and practice communication and negotiation skills with each other.

When conducting an all-day retreat, be sure to address the following challenges:

- Have enough chaperons. A good ratio is 1 adult for every 4 youth.

- Be sure the chaperons have a relationship with the youth so that youth will listen to them.

- Provide plenty of recreational activities along with the educational ones so that youth have structured time to release energy.

- If you invite a speaker, it is important to know what she or he will say in advance to ensure it will be an appropriate message for the youth.

How should I end the program?

If time and money allows, it's nice to bring closure with a graduation ceremony. In the original program, youth invited their parents for a celebration in which they received certificates and refreshments were served.

Where can I get free supplies?

"Professional begging" is an excellent way to obtain supplies. Ask local stores, companies, restaurants and factories to donate needed items. See the Resource Section for tips and a sample letter for soliciting donations.

There are also agencies that supply free condoms and HIV information pamphlets:

CDC National Prevention Information Network
Post Office Box 6003
Rockville, Maryland 20849-6003
1-800-458-5231

Tips on Facilitating

▼ **Make sure you have a comfortable, private space** for the group to meet.

▼ **Stand where everyone can see you.** A semicircle works well for the group.

▼ **Watch the time:**

- Know how much time you want to devote to each activity.

- Be careful of conversations getting off track. Help guide youth back to the task at hand.

- Try to limit interruptions (phone calls, recreation center business, etc.).

▼ **Be aware of your audience.** Are they looking bored? Do they need a break? Do they understand what you are saying? Are they offended/scared/overwhelmed by what you are saying?

▼ **Be FIRED UP!!!!** Attitude is everything! Keep your voice exciting, use body language, walk around when you talk—keep them listening!

▼ **Get to know names** of the youth and use them.

▼ **Make sure everyone is participating.** Don't call on the same people all the time. Try to help more reserved youth join in the discussions.

▼ **Integrate previous lessons** when applicable. (*Example:* What else might Tavon want to think about while he makes his decision? How about his values? Remember when we talked about values last week? How would values be important when you are making a decision?)

▼ **Keep it interactive.** Don't lecture too much. (For example, when discussing invulnerability do not define it right away, instead ask the group participants to define it.)

▼ **When youth are in small groups** make sure you go around and check in with each group.

▼ **Use examples often** when explaining things.

▼ **Define words** you aren't sure everyone knows (or have youth define them) as you go along.

▼ **Remain flexible.** If you don't have time to finish a session, you can go overtime, add a session, or skip some of the games. You do not need to be rigid with the curriculum.

▼ **Remember,** many of the above tips are easier to implement if you have 2 group leaders who are able to work well together.

Tips on Managing Behavior

Behavior is a form of communication. When a youth misbehaves or breaks one of the rules agreed upon by the group, that youth is communicating something to the group and the group leaders.

The message could be anything, ranging from "I don't understand the rule" to "I'm bored" to "This topic is embarrassing, and I have to move the focus off me" to "I'm being ignored and I want more attention." There are endless possible messages, and numerous responses available to facilitators.

Rules

▼ You and the group should define the rules everyone agrees to follow. (See Session 1, Activity 4 on groundrules.)

▼ These rules should help to guide youths' behavior, and will give you a framework for addressing behaviors and consequences.

Reinforcements

▼ Use frequent opportunities to reinforce youth for what they are doing RIGHT. In other words, catch them being good! Some youth may not be used to praise and might feel uncomfortable at first, especially if they get teased by other youth, or interpret it as being singled out.

▼ Remember that praise can be given verbally, nonverbally or tangibly (openly or discreetly). See page 19 for more tips on using reinforcements.

Verbal Reinforcement

• Youth can be verbally reinforced for behaviors or things they do: "That's a good point." "It was very considerate when you shared your materials." "You must feel proud of yourself for getting such good grades." "I really like the way you're sitting—it shows that you're paying attention."

Nonverbal Reinforcement

- Attention and recognition can be given in very subtle and in unobtrusive ways. A look, a smile, a touch on the shoulder or a handshake are all ways of acknowledging another individual without saying a word or calling attention to that person.

- Nonverbal reinforcement can be very useful if you notice that someone is beginning to drift from the group's activities or needs to be brought back into the group. It is particularly effective for the second group leader to use, since it doesn't disrupt the verbal flow of the group or the material being presented by the other group leader.

- You may choose to start off by pairing a nonverbal reinforcer with a verbal one (e.g., shake someone's hand while saying, "I like the way you acted out that character in the roleplay").

- Later, if you use just the nonverbal, the youth will be able to associate it with the verbal statement you made earlier.

Tangible Rewards

- Some people like to use tangible rewards, such as raisins, M&M's, or paper tokens, which can later be traded in for a small prize.

- Rewards can become expensive, or, in the case of tokens, require some planning.

Consequences

- Have youth participate in defining the consequences as well as the rewards for their actions. That way, no one will be surprised when a consequence is implemented.

- Make sure that consequences are reasonable. Youth tend to be *very* strict with themselves when talking about consequences in more abstract terms. (*Example:* "We should kick him out of the group for 2 sessions and then his mother has to bring him back in.")

- Be realistic and choose consequences you are likely and willing to implement.

Commands

▼ Commands are ways of letting youth know what you expect of them. They are most effective if they have been discussed beforehand, so that everyone knows the expectations.

▼ Commands should be short and to the point. Sometimes parents make the mistake of giving a string of commands at one time (e.g., "Go upstairs, wash your hands, pick up your clothes, do your homework, then come downstairs and fix the hamburgers.") and then get upset when kids, particularly younger ones, only do the first or the last command. Kids are more likely to follow rules that they understand, so be brief and to the point.

▼ Always remember to reinforce a youth for following your command. See page 18 for more information on using commands.

Ignoring Behavior

▼ Sometimes, the most effective thing to do is simply to ignore certain behaviors. If a youth is doing something that is relatively harmless to the group process, ignore it, and reinforce someone else in the group for something he or she is doing right.

▼ Continue to monitor the first youth's behavior. As soon as he or she does something right, reinforce for what was just done.

▼ **Do not get into a power struggle with youth. You are the adult and the person in charge, so you always have options. There is never a need to put a youth down.**

Time-Outs

▼ Although time-outs are most often used with younger kids, variations can also be used with adolescents. For example, a youth may be asked to step out of the group for 5 minutes if she/he is being disruptive of the group process and does not seem to be able to change the behavior.

▼ Again, time-outs are something that should be discussed with youth beforehand so that everyone understands the expectations.

▼ During time-outs, youth should not leave the area, but should stand immediately outside the group or group room. No one, including the facilitators, should talk to a youth during a time-out, since this is not a time for attention.

▼ If the youth continues to act out, the time-out may need to be extended.

▼ Once the 5 minutes (or number of minutes given) are up, the youth should be brought back into the group.

▼ Take advantage of the first opportunity to catch the youth being good. Remember that this youth needs an opportunity to save face, be readmitted into the group process and make amends.

▼ Do not continue to talk to a youth about the misbehavior after a time-out. If further discussion is necessary, do it at a later time.

Planned Breaks

▼ Plan to take a break about halfway through the session. Two hours can be a very long time to sit in a group, especially if youth have already been sitting in a classroom all day long.

▼ Usually, it works well to save any snacks to have during the break, so that snacks become reinforcers for having accomplished the tasks of the first half of the session.

▼ The group's behavior may indicate they are ready for a break before the planned time, especially if they are feeling tired, bored or lacking energy.

▼ Sometimes, a youth may ask for a break. If you think it is a reasonable request, reinforce that youth for being self-aware and give the group a minute to stretch.

Feedback

▼ Be open to feedback and attentive to what your audience is telling you.

▼ Youth may have suggestions about activities, preferences and dislikes, which may actually make the group more enjoyable for everyone.

Positive Limit Setting

▼ Part of establishing autonomy is testing limits. Know that youth may be likely to test your limits.

▼ Try to remain positive. There are so many Don'ts in the world, especially for kids, so try to emphasize the Do's.

▼ For example, when youth are first defining the rules of the group, help them phrase things in a positive way—I will respect the opinions of other members of the group—rather than negatively—No making fun of other people's opinions.

Taking a Youth Aside

▼ Sometimes, you may notice that a youth is preoccupied or withdrawn, or acting out in an uncharacteristic way. Without reinforcing the behavior, you still have the option to take that youth aside to talk individually while the other group leader continues to work with the rest of the group.

▼ This may be the best way to get at what is on the youth's mind, and may be quite relevant to something being discussed in that session.

▼ Make yourself available to talk after group, if necessary.

▼ Coordinate with the other group leader beforehand so you both understand what is taking place when you walk out of the room with a youth and leave the other group leader alone with the group for a while.

Using Commands

■ State your command clearly and succinctly: "Please sit down."

■ State your command again, followed by a statement of the consequence for noncompliance: "Please sit down. If you don't sit down, I will stop the video."

■ If the youth complies, reinforce him/her for following the group rules: "Thank you."

■ If the youth does not comply, follow through on the consequence: Stop the video. Then, give the command again: "Please sit down."

■ If the youth complies this time, reinforce him/her and continue with the activity. If the youth does not comply, let him/her know that you will give a time out: "Please sit down. If you do not sit down, you will take a time out."

■ If the youth complies, reinforce him/her. If he/she doesn't comply, give a time-out: "You need to go to time-out for 5 minutes."

Make sure that consequences are reasonable and match the degree of the misbehavior. Never threaten a youth with a consequence that you are not willing to follow through on. It will put you in a corner and detract from your credibility.

Instead of Punishment

1. **Point out a way to be helpful.** "Instead of playing with the paper, I'd like you to help me collect everyone's papers."

2. **Express your feelings strongly, without attacking character.** "I'm upset that I am constantly interrupted, and I can't finish telling this story."

3. **State your expectations.** "I expect that group members will express their thoughts to the whole group rather than carry on private conversations."

4. **Show the youth how to make amends.** "The popcorn scattered all over the floor will need to be picked up before we go on to the next activity."

5. **Give the youth a choice.** "You can either remain in your seat and participate, or you can leave the room until we've completed the discussion."

6. **Take action.** "Since the group is not following direction, we will stop this video."

7. **Problem solve.** "How can we make sure that no more juice gets spilled?"

8. **Allow the youth to experience consequences for the behavior.** "Since you are unable to stop disrupting the group, you need to be in time-out for the next 5 minutes."

Adapted from A. Faber and E. Mazlish. 1995. *How to Talk So Kids Will Listen and Listen So Kids Will Talk.* New York: Simon and Schuster Audio.

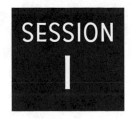

SESSION 1

Trust Building and Group Cohesion

Purpose	Youth will establish a cohesive group, set groundrules and begin learning skills for decision making.

Session Overview
(100 minutes)

1 Introduction Game

- Option A: Flying Objects **OLDER YOUTH** (10 minutes)

- Option B: Double Letter **YOUNGER YOUTH** (10 minutes)

2 *Focus on Kids* **Program Overview** (15 minutes)

3 Group Cohesion Activity

- Option A: Burning Buildings **OLDER YOUTH** (15 minutes)

- Option B: Human Knot **YOUNGER YOUTH** (15 minutes)

4 Establishing Groundrules (20 minutes)

5 Family Tree (20 minutes)

6 SODA Decision-Making Model: Step 1 (15 minutes)

7 Wrap-Up and Closing Ritual (5 minutes)

Preparation

Pre-Session Activities

❏ Confirm space and time.

❏ Call youth and remind them and their families about meeting.

❏ Prepare snacks.

❏ Read over and become familiar with Session 1 activities.

❏ Review the Family Tree stories and modify if necessary for your target community.

❏ Become familiar with the Family Tree to be able to tell the story without reading from the sheet.

❏ Make SODA Decision-Making Model chart. (See Sample on page 48.)

Materials

❏ snacks

❏ newsprint

❏ posterboard for Family Tree, Groundrules and SODA Model charts

❏ markers

❏ masking tape

❏ 3 soft, silly objects for Flying Objects activity (e.g., roll of toilet paper, stuffed animal, etc.) **OLDER YOUTH**

❏ 2 boards for Burning Buildings activity (1' x 8' wood planks) OR masking tape to make lines on the floor to represent planks **OLDER YOUTH**

❏ Question Box (A shoe box and materials for youth to decorate it.)

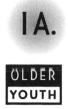

IA.

OLDER YOUTH

Introduction Game: Flying Objects

Source: Adapted from Center for Experiential Education, Boulder, Colorado.

😊 **Objective:**	Youth will build group cohesion.
🕐 **Time:**	10 minutes
✂ **Materials:**	3 soft, silly objects that are easy to throw (roll of toilet paper, stuffed animal, etc.)

Procedure

1 Have group members stand in a circle.

2 Begin by calling out a person's name and then throwing her or him the first object. Direct that person to choose someone else, say this person's name and throw the object to her or him.

3 Continue until you have done 1 complete round, with everyone in the group receiving the object (no one should get it more than once), and the object has come back to you. Explain that the game requires people to remember whom they threw the object to, so they can throw the object to the same person for several more rotations.

4 Begin again by throwing the first object. Before it has completed the cycle, start the pattern again with object 2. Then add object 3. Continue, using all 3 objects. Try to keep all 3 objects in rotation for 3 rotations.

Notes for Group Leaders: This activity works well with a group of 5-12 people. If you have more than 15 people, divide into 2 groups.

This group-building activity helps the group leader learn the youths' names and helps youth learn to work together and build a sense of a group.

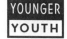

1B.

YOUNGER
YOUTH

Introduction Game: Double Letter

Source: Planned Parenthood of Maryland's STARS (Students Talking About Responsible Sexuality).

☺ **Objective:**   Youth will be able to call each other by name.

🕐 **Time:**   10 minutes

✂ **Materials:**   None

Procedure

1 Have youth sit in a circle.

2 Ask youth to think of an adjective that begins with the first letter of their name, e.g., Devilish Diedre or Awesome Anthony (this is a double letter name). They must keep this name to themselves until it is their turn to share with the group.

3 Begin by asking the person to your right to say his or her double letter name. Then introduce yourself by your double letter name and re-introduce the person to your right. The person to the left of the group leader then introduces him/herself, re-introduces the group leader, then re-introduces the person on the right of the group leader.
(*Note:* If there are a lot of youth and they are quite young you can limit re-introductions to the previous 2 individuals.)

4 Continue this process until everyone is introduced. Instruct group members not to help each other; only the person being introduced may assist the introducer.

Notes for Group Leaders: This activity works best with younger youth. It is an effective group-building activity because it helps the group leaders learn youths' names and helps youth learn to work together and build a sense of a group.

2.

Focus On Kids
Program Overview

☺ **Objective:** Youth will learn about the *Focus on Kids* program, and will establish a group name and opening and closing rituals.

🕐 **Time:** 15 minutes

✂ **Materials:** Newsprint and markers

Procedure

1 Explain that the *Focus on Kids* program will last for 8 sessions, and that to "graduate" youth must be present for at least 6 sessions. In the first 6 sessions they will learn information about decision making; values; how to get information; communication skills; negotiation skills; goals for the future; and facts about sex, teen pregnancy, STD, HIV, drug use and drug selling.

In the last 2 sessions, they will review what they've learned and plan a project to teach others. Possible projects include writing raps, performing skits for other youth or community residents, making posters, or holding a meeting to teach others about making decisions.

Optional: If you are using the all-day retreat option for Session 6, tell youth about the retreat and what day it will be held. Explain that they will need to attend at least 3 sessions to qualify to go on the retreat.

2 Explain that this is the youths' group and they need to come up with the following:

• a group name

• an opening ritual—something they will start each group meeting with (e.g., juice and popcorn, a prayer, sharing something about their week, a game, etc.)

- a closing ritual—some way to end the session (e.g., wrapping up what they have learned, a prayer, cleaning up, etc.)

- groundrules

3 For now, have the youth come up with a group name and rituals. Explain that after the next game, they can begin to work on the groundrules.

Notes for Group Leaders: If youth are having trouble coming up with a name or opening and closing rituals, give them some time to think about it. You can brainstorm for now and then vote on the name and rituals the following week.

These are important components of group cohesion, so the group leaders should encourage youth to make a choice and should be sure to incorporate their choices.

3A.

Group Cohesion Activity: Burning Buildings

Source: Adapted from Center for Experiential Education, Boulder, Colorado.

☺ **Objective:**   Youth will build group cohesion by achieving a common goal.

🕐 **Time:**   15 minutes

✂ **Materials:**   Two 1' x 8' wood planks, or masking tape to make lines on the floor to represent planks

---

Procedure

1 Put the 2 wood planks together end to end to form a 16' beam. Have half the youth stand on one end and the other half stand on the other end (see diagram below). Tell them they are on the 86th floor of the Twin Towers in New York City.

Half of them are trapped in one of the towers and there is a fire raging behind them. The other half are firefighters, who have to save the first group and make it to the other side to fight the fire. They have to switch sides without falling off the beam. Any time any individual falls off they have to start the game all over.

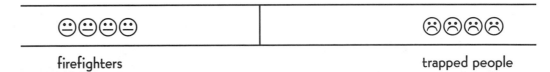

☺☺☺☺	☹☹☹☹
firefighters	trapped people

2 Have youth work out a solution. Allow approximately 10 minutes.

3 After youth have managed to switch sides on the plank, lead a discussion about the activity using the following questions:

- How did you figure it out?

- What worked as a group to help you reach your goal?

- What didn't work?

- Who was the leader?

- How did you all reach agreement?

Emphasize that this game shows how important it is to listen to each other and work as a team.

Notes for Group Leaders: Most youth love this game! Boys often have more trouble with it because they do not want to touch each other. They may need to be told it is OK to touch each other.

If your group is larger than 10–15, ask for volunteers to participate.

3B.

YOUNGER YOUTH

Group Cohesion Activity: Human Knot

Source: Planned Parenthood of Maryland's STARS (Students Talking About Responsible Sexuality).

☺ **Objective:** Youth will build group cohesion by working together to achieve a common goal.

🕐 **Time:** 15 minutes

✂ **Materials:** None

Procedure

1 Ask youth to stand in a circle. Have them reach out with their right hands and join hands with a person who is across from them (not next to them). Then have them reach out with their left hands and join hands with a different person across from them. When everyone is holding hands, the group has formed the human knot.

2 Direct the group to untangle the knot without letting go of hands. The untangled knot will take the form of a circle, with some people facing into the circle and others facing away from it.

3 After youth have untangled the knot, discuss the activity using the following questions:

- How did you figure it out?

- What worked to help the group reach the goal of untying the knot?

- What didn't work?

- Who was the leader?

- How did you all reach agreement?

Emphasize that this game shows how important it is to listen to each other and work as a team.

Notes for Group Leaders: Both older and younger youth seem to really enjoy this. If there is trouble untangling, have them start a hand squeeze. One person squeezes the hand of the person he or she is holding, who in turn squeezes the hand of the next person. The squeeze should go through the whole circle. If a participant's hand is never squeezed, there are 2 circles, and the knot can only be undone into 2 circles.

4.

Establishing Groundrules

Source: Adapted from Center for Population Options' Guide to Implementing TAP (Teens for AIDS Prevention Peer Education Program).

☺ **Objective:** Youth will establish an agreed-upon, appropriate code of behavior for the group.

🕐 **Time:** 20 minutes

✂ **Materials:** Posterboard and markers

Question Box (or envelopes)

☑ **Preparation:** Review **Suggested Groundrules** and be familiar with them. (See page 33.)

Procedure

1 Explain that because the group will discuss sensitive issues, youth should agree upon groundrules. Ask the group to suggest groundrules that will help them be more comfortable discussing sensitive topics. List suggestions on the posterboard (or ask for a volunteer to do the writing).

After youth have generated some rules, propose the rules from the **Suggested Groundrules** list. Make sure the youth agree to all the rules that the group finally adopts.

2 Have each youth and group leader sign the posterboard with the rules.

3 Keep this posterboard in the room throughout the sessions and refer to it often. Eventually, youth will remind each other when some behavior becomes counter-productive to the group process.

4 Introduce the anonymous Question Box. You or the youth can decorate a shoe box or similar box and put a slot in the top for people to anonymously slip in questions and comments. Find an appropriate spot where the box will not be tampered with and where youth can put

a question in without anyone seeing them.

You could also give each youth an envelope addressed to your work address, and have envelopes available at each meeting to encourage youth to mail anonymous questions to you.

Suggested Groundrules

Respect

Give your undivided attention to the person who is speaking.

Confidentiality

Keep personal information that we share in this group in this room. But it is OK to share factual information about HIV, drugs, birth control or STD with others.

Openness

Be open and honest, but do not tell about others' (family, neighbors, friends) personal/private lives. It is OK to discuss general situations as examples, but don't use names, or say things that would let people identify the individuals. (*Note*: This is a very important point that must be on the list.)

Nonjudgmental approach

Disagree with another person's point of view or behaviors, but do not judge or put down another person.

Nondiscrimination

Be aware that members in the group have different backgrounds and different sexual orientations. Be careful about insensitive remarks regarding this diversity.

Right to pass

It is always OK to pass, to say "I'd rather not do this activity" or "I don't think I want to answer that question."

Anonymity

It is OK to ask a question anonymously if desired. You can use the Question Box.

Acceptance

It is OK to feel uncomfortable; even adults feel uncomfortable when they talk about sensitive and personal topics like sexuality or HIV.

Responsibility

Come to the session and be on time. If you cannot attend, notify another group member or a group leader.

5. Family Tree

Source: Adapted from R. N. Ford, W. H. Gregory and J. Mariweather. 1993. The MBF Model of Identity for "He": My Baby's Father. FAJR Associates.

☺ **Objective:** Youth will be able to explain that decision making occurs in a social context.

Youth will be able to talk about their lives without disclosing personal information.

Youth will understand that decisions made while they are young can have an impact on their future.

🕐 **Time:** 20 minutes

✂ **Materials:** Posterboard and markers

☑ **Preparation:** Become familiar with the Family Tree stories and diagrams. (See pages 36–45.)

You might need to adapt the Family Tree for your target community. This should be done with community leaders. (See Getting Started, page 7, for information on adapting the program.)

Notes for Group Leaders: The family tree is used to teach youth that decision making occurs in a social context. Our family, culture and values affect how we make decisions. The family tree is also used to allow youth to share their feelings without disclosing private information.

This curriculum includes 2 versions of the family tree, but it should be adapted for your audience. The family tree diagram should reflect an average family in your community and some of the individuals who influence youth in both a positive and negative way. Name the characters with popular names from your community.

Remember that, although you will adapt the story, it should be *youth-driven*. Give youth the skeleton of the story and have them fill in the details of the characters and their relationships.

Procedure

1 Have youth sit in a semicircle. Tell them that you have a story and want their help in telling it. Explain that, in this story, female symbols ♀ represent women and male symbols ♂ represent men.

Explain as you go along what the connecting lines mean:

- double lines mean 2 people are married

- dotted lines represent children

- single solid lines indicate a relationship between 2 people who are not married

Put the characters on the posterboard as you talk about them. (See diagram on page 38.)

2 Tell the story. Story 1 takes place in an urban environment. Story 2 takes place in a suburban environment. Choose the story that best fits the group.

3 Help youth fill in the details of the characters and their relationships by asking the discussion questions for the appropriate story. (*Note:* There are different discussion questions for girls and boys. If you have a mixed group, ask some questions from both sets. Record details in your notes to refer to in future discussions.)

4 Summarize by reminding youth that every day we must make decisions that are going to affect the rest of our lives. Sometimes we don't decide what will happen to us, we just let whatever happens happen. Tell them they will be talking about a way to make decisions that gives them more control about what is going to happen in their lives. Then, using the next activity, introduce the SODA Decision-Making Model.

Notes for Group Leaders: There should be a short make-up session for any youth who miss the Family Tree activity, scheduled as soon as possible— for example, the half hour before or after the next session.

Story 1—Urban Version

Note: Refer to the diagrams on page 38 as you tell the story.

I want to introduce you to Tavon and Chantel who are _____ years old (use the average age of youth in the group). I want you to meet their brothers and sisters and cousins, as well as the rest of their family.

Right now Tavon and Chantel live with their grandmother, mother, mother's husband, a brother, a sister, an aunt (mother's sister) and a cousin. But let's start by going back about 16 years and learning more about Tavon and Chantel's family.

One Saturday night, Mary meets Al at a party at her girlfriend's house. Al is 20 years old and he looks good. He and Mary spend a lot of time together at the party. Al starts to visit Mary at her house, although Mary's mother, Esther (Tavon and Chantel's grandmother) says Mary needs to spend more time on her homework and less time with Al.

After a while, Mary starts going over to Al's house. Al lives with his grandmother and 2 older cousins. Mary and Al are alone there quite a bit. It isn't too long before Al and Mary start to have sex. Two months later, Mary finds out she is pregnant. Mary has a little boy—this little boy is Tavon.

(Draw diagram 1 on the posterboard as you tell this part of the story.)

Mary sees less of Al after Tavon is born, although Al comes by with gifts sometimes. Mary goes back to school, so Mary's mother, Esther, takes care of Tavon most of the time.

One evening Mary is hanging with some friends and she meets John. John has a car, and he invites Mary to go riding with him. Mary likes John and agrees to go with him. John and Mary date for a couple of years and during that time Mary becomes pregnant again and has a little girl—Chantel. After a couple of years John and Mary break up and John moves to a town several hours away.

(Add John and Chantel to the Family Tree. See diagram 2.)

David is an old friend of Mary's and Mary has known him for many years. David is 25 years old, and he works in a construction company. David recently moved out of the house he was sharing with his girlfriend, Yvonne, and their child, Brian (age 7). David and Mary start seeing each other. In about a year, they get married.

Two years later, Tamika is born; and a year later Cory is born. David and Mary have their own apartment, and Tavon who still lives with his Grandmother, Esther, starts to spend weekends with them. David's son, Brian, lives with his mother, Yvonne.

(Add David, Tamika, Cory, Yvonne and Brian to the Family Tree. See diagram 3.)

Let's move to the present. David and Mary have moved back in with Mary's mother, Esther, because David lost his construction job last year. Mary's sister Ebony (Tavon and Chantel's aunt) and her 2-year-old son Omar are also living with Esther.

(Add Ebony and Omar to the Family Tree. See diagram 4. Review who is living in the house—Esther, Ebony, Omar, Mary, David, Tamika, Cory, Tavon and Chantel. Put in the ages of the children at the present time—Chantel and Tavon should be close to the ages of the youth in the group.)

Family Tree Diagrams
Story 1 — Urban Version

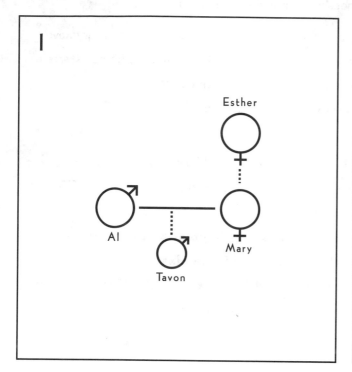

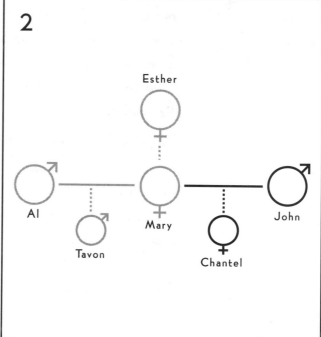

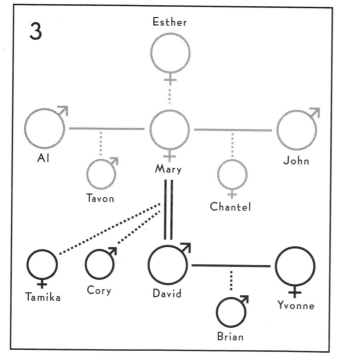

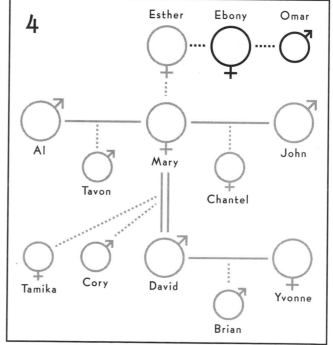

(*Note:* Final Family Tree Chart will look like diagram 4.)

Discussion Questions Story 1—Urban Version

Questions for Boys

- What can you tell me about Tavon?

  - What does he do in his spare time?

  - How is he doing in school?

- What can you tell me about Chantel? (Continue with a few other characters.)

- What can you tell me about Tavon's relationship with other relatives, both inside and outside of the household?

  - Does Tavon see his father, Al? How does he feel about him?

  - How did he feel when his mother married David?

  - How does he feel about Cory?

  - How does he feel about his mother?

  - How does he feel about his grandmother, Esther?

  - Does David still see his other child, Brian?

  - How does Tavon feel about David's other child?

  - How does Mary feel about Yvonne?

- Whom does Tavon talk to when he has a problem?

- What does he do after school?

- What are Tavon's friends like? Does he have a girlfriend?

- What does he want to do when he is grown up?

- What kinds of decisions does Tavon have to make? What kinds of decisions does the family have to make?

- Are the decisions Tavon is making now going to allow him to do what he wants to do when he grows up?

Questions for Girls

- What can you tell me about Chantel?

  - What does she do in her spare time?

  - How is she doing in school?

- What can you tell me about Tavon? (Continue with a few other characters.)

- What can you tell me about Chantel's relationship with other relatives, both inside and outside of the household?

  - Does Chantel see her father, John? How does she feel about him?

  - How did she feel when her mother married David?

  - How does she feel about Tamika?

  - How does she feel about her mother?

  - How does she feel about her grandmother, Esther?

  - Does David still see his other child, Brian?

  - How does Chantel feel about David's other child?

  - How does Mary feel about Yvonne?

- Whom does Chantel talk to when she has a problem?

- What does she do after school?

- What are her friends like? Does she have a boyfriend?

- What does she want to do when she is grown up?

- What kinds of decisions does Chantel have to make? What kinds of decisions does the family have to make?

- Are the decisions Chantel is making now going to allow her to do what she wants to do when she grows up?

Story 2—Suburban Version

Note: Refer to the diagrams on page 43 as you tell the story.

I want to introduce you to Randy and Kim who are _____ years old (use the average age of youth in the group). I want you to meet their parents and half-brothers as well as the rest of their family.

Right now Randy and Kim are living with their mother and spend every other weekend with their father, his new wife and their 2 sons (Randy and Kim's half-brothers). But let's start by going back about 16 years and learning more about Randy and Kim's family.

About 20 years ago, Nadine (Randy and Kim's mother) is 20 years old and in her second year of college. Nadine and Ralph have been going out for 2 years, ever since Nadine started college. Ralph is graduating this year and has taken a job in another state. They decide to get married so they can stay together.

Ralph takes the job and they plan for Nadine to finish her education at another college nearby and then work so that Ralph can go to medical school and become a doctor. But the first year they are married Nadine gets pregnant and has to drop out of school.

After Randy is born, Ralph stays at the job he is at instead of going to med school. Nadine works occasionally but most of the time stays home with Randy. Two years later they have another child, Kim.

(Draw diagram 1 while you are telling this part of the story.)

When Randy is 10 and Kim is 8, Nadine and Ralph have begun to fight a lot. Nadine is angry that Ralph is never home. He leaves early in the morning and does not come home until late at night. He often has to work weekends too. The fighting gets worse, and one night Ralph and Nadine talk to Randy and Kim and tell them that they have decided to separate. Randy and Kim will live with their mother and see their father on weekends.

A year later Ralph and Nadine divorce. Later that year, Ralph tells Randy and Kim that he is marrying Jeanie.

(Draw a line through the equal sign between Ralph and Nadine and add in Jeanie. See diagram 2.)

One year later, Joshua is born. Then, a few months ago, Ralph and Jeanie had their second son, Michael.

(Draw in Joshua and Michael. See diagram 3.)

Let's move to the present. Randy and Kim are _____ (use the average age of youth in the group). Nadine has just started dating a new man named Sam. She seems to really like him and is much happier these days. Ralph and Jeanie have been talking about moving to another town that is 45 minutes away.

(Draw Sam in the diagram and put in ages of youth. See diagram 4.)

Family Tree Diagrams
Story 2 – Suburban Version

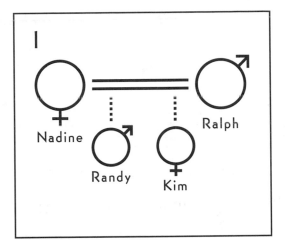

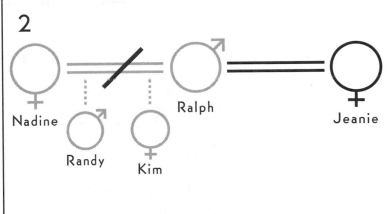

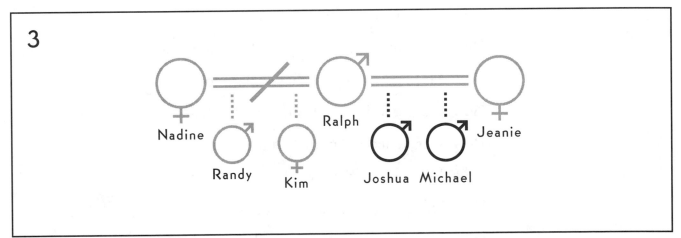

(*Note:* Final Family Tree Chart will look like diagram 4.)

Discussion Questions
Story 2—Suburban Version

Questions for Boys

- What can you tell me about Randy?

  - What does he do in his spare time?

  - How is he doing in school?

- What can you tell me about Kim? (Continue with other characters.)

- What can you tell me about Randy's relationship with other relatives, both inside and outside of the household?

  - What was the divorce like for him?

  - How often does Randy see his father? How does he feel about him?

  - How did he feel when his father married Jeanie?

  - How does he feel about Joshua and Michael?

  - How does he feel about his mother?

  - How does he feel about Sam?

  - How does Nadine feel about Jeanie?

- Whom does Randy talk to when he has a problem?

- What does he do after school?

- What are Randy's friends like? Does he have a girlfriend?

- What does he want to do when he is grown up?

- What kinds of decisions does Randy have to make? What kinds of decisions does the family have to make?

- Are the decisions Randy is making now going to allow him to do what he wants to do when he grows up?

Questions for Girls

- What can you tell me about Kim?

  - What does she do in her spare time?

  - How is she doing in school?

- What can you tell me about Randy. (Continue with other characters.)

- What can you tell me about Kim's relationship with other relatives, both inside and outside of the household?

  - What was the divorce like for her?

  - How often does Kim see her father? How does she feel about him?

  - How did she feel when her father married Jeanie?

  - How does she feel about Joshua and Michael?

  - How does she feel about her mother?

  - How does she feel about Sam?

  - How does Nadine feel about Jeanie?

- Whom does Kim talk to when she has a problem?

- What does she do after school?

- What are Kim's friends like? Does she have a boyfriend?

- What does she want to do when she is grown up?

- What kinds of decisions does Kim have to make? What kinds of decisions does the family have to make?

- Are the decisions Kim is making now going to allow her to do what she wants to do when she grows up?

6. SODA Decision-Making Model—Step 1: Stop

Source: S. Schinke, A. Gordon and R. Weston. 1990. Self-Instruction to Prevent HIV Infection Among African-American and Hispanic-American Adolescents. Journal of Consulting and Clinical Psychology 58 (4): 432-436.

☺ **Objective:** Youth will learn decision making, with a focus on Step 1: Stop and state the problem.

🕐 **Time:** 15 minutes

✂ **Materials:** Posterboard and markers to make a SODA Model chart (See sample.) *Note:* Use this chart at each session.

Procedure

1 Briefly introduce the following steps of decision making.

Step 1: Stop—**Stop and state the problem.** Pause and give yourself time to decide what the problem really is.

Step 2: Options—**Consider the options** or choices and the consequences of those choices. Educate yourself so you know all the choices and consequences before you make a decision.

Step 3: Decide—**Decide and choose the best solution** from the options. What is best will vary depending on the problem and your values (strongly held beliefs). Making a decision is done by weighing the advantages and disadvantages of the options.

Step 4: Action—**Act on your decision.** Once a decision is made, it must be put into action. To accomplish this, you may need to learn new skills for communication, negotiation or other skills related to carrying out the decision (e.g., condom use, use of birth control).

2 Explain that today's lesson will concentrate on the **Stop** step. Explain that first a person must recognize and define a problem or a decision that needs to be made. **Illustrate this process using an example from the Family Tree**.

YOUNGER YOUTH

Example for younger youth: It is raining. Chantel gets ready for school wearing her new tennis shoes. Her Mom tells her to put on her old shoes, and they get into a fight.

Stop!: What is the problem?

What is the problem from Chantel's point of view?

What is the problem from her Mom's point of view?

OLDER YOUTH

Example for older youth: Tavon wants to play basketball during 8th period. His mother wants him to take advanced math. Tavon's girlfriend wants to take English with him. Tavon's adviser thinks he should consider remedial English.

Stop!: What is the problem?

What is the problem from Tavon's point of view?

What is the problem from his Mom's point of view?

3 Ask youth to give an example of a recent decision and identify what problem they were trying to solve.

Notes for Group Leaders: To prevent boredom during this discussion, keep the pace fast and make it as interactive as possible.

Sample Chart

Decision Making

Stop
. . Stop and state the problem.

Options
. . Consider the options or choices and
the consequences of those choices.

Decide
. . Decide and choose the best solution.

Action
. . Act on your decision.

7.

Wrap-Up and Closing Ritual

☺ **Objective:** Youth will provide feedback on Session 1 and summarize what they have learned.

🕑 **Time:** 5 minutes

✂ **Materials:** None

Procedure

1 Have the group sit in a circle. Discuss what they would like to do as a closing ritual. If they don't come up with one, suggest something (e.g., a hand squeeze or special wave).

2 Explain that you also want some feedback during the closing ritual.

Ask youth the following questions:

- What did they like?

- What didn't they like?

- What did they learn?

- What would they like to learn more about at another session?

3 Remind youth of the next meeting time and place. Tell them to remind each other. Offer to call the night before the meeting to remind them of it.

4 Provide a way for youth to contact you if they need to. Also remind them that they can put questions in the Question Box during the week.

Risks and Values

Purpose	Youth will understand why they may feel invulnerable and how this can place them at risk for HIV/STD or unplanned pregnancy.
	Youth will learn to identify their values and use them to make decisions.

Session Overview
(105 minutes)

1 Opening Ritual and Review (10 minutes)

2 How Risky Is It? (15 minutes)

3 What Are You Concerned About? (10 minutes)

4 Why Do People Feel Invulnerable? (10 minutes)

5 Defining a Value (5 minutes)

6 Rank Your Values (20 minutes)

7 Values Voting (20–60 minutes)

8 What Youth Can Do (10 minutes)

9 Wrap-Up and Closing Ritual (5 minutes)

Preparation

Pre-Session Activities

- ❑ Read over and become familiar with Session 2 activities.

- ❑ Prepare Snacks.

- ❑ Copy **Rank Your Values** worksheet for each participant. (See page 66.)

- ❑ Make How Risky Is It? signs: "Stop!—Risky!," "Use Caution," "Safe—Go Ahead." (See samples on pages 57–59.)

- ❑ Make "Agree" and "Disagree" signs for values voting. (See samples on pages 70 and 71.)

Materials

- ❑ snacks

- ❑ Family Tree, SODA Model and Groundrules charts

- ❑ masking tape

- ❑ newsprint

- ❑ markers

- ❑ **Rank Your Values** worksheet, 1 for each participant

- ❑ scissors, 1 for each participant

- ❑ clear tape, 1 roll for each 5–6 participants

- ❑ colored 8-1/2" x 11" paper, 1 piece for each participant

- ❑ signs for How Risky Is It? activity

- ❑ "Agree" and "Disagree" signs

- ❑ List of **Values Voting Items** (See page 69.)

1. Opening Ritual and Review

☺ **Objective:**	Youth will review highlights from Session 1.
⏰ **Time:**	10 minutes
✂ **Materials:**	Groundrules, SODA Model and Family Tree charts

Procedure

1 After the opening ritual, sit down with youth and remind them of groundrules. Have any new members sign the rules once they agree.

2 Answer any questions that have been put in the Question Box.

3 Ask youth to tell you what each letter in SODA stands for.

Step 1: Stop—**Stop and state the problem.** Pause and give yourself time to decide what the problem really is.

Step 2: Options—**Consider the options** or choices and the consequences of those choices. Educate yourself so you know all the choices and consequences before you make a decision.

Step 3: Decide—**Decide and choose the best solution** from the options. What is best will vary depending on the problem and your values (strongly held beliefs). Making a decision is done by weighing the advantages and disadvantages of the options.

Step 4: Action—**Act on your decision.** Once a decision is made, it must be put into action. To accomplish this, you may need to learn new skills for communication, negotiation or other skills related to carrying out the decision (e.g., condom use, use of birth control).

4 Ask youth to briefly tell newcomers about characters from the Family Tree activity. Show the Family Tree chart to reinforce what they share.

2. How Risky Is It?

☺ **Objective:** Youth will identify behaviors that do and do not put them at risk for HIV infection.

🕐 **Time:** 15 minutes

✂ **Materials:** Signs with the headings "Stop!—Risky!" "Use Caution," and "Safe—Go Ahead" placed at different places around the room (See samples.)

Procedure

1 Tell youth that this activity will help them understand which behaviors place them at risk for HIV infection and which behaviors do not. Explain that you will read a behavior from a list and they should stand by the sign that reflects the level of risk for HIV infection they believe the behavior represents.

2 Read the following list of behaviors one at a time. Have youth move to stand by the appropriate sign. After each behavior is decided upon, ask: Why is this behavior risky or not risky? (*Note*: Be sure youth have the correct information before moving to the next behavior.)

Behaviors

- Not having sexual intercourse (abstinence) (*Safe*)

- Using a public toilet (*Safe*)

- Sharing needles to inject drugs (*Stop*)

- French kissing (*Caution*)

- Anal intercourse (*Stop*)

- Shaking hands with a person who has AIDS (*Safe*)

- Being born to a mother with HIV (*Caution*)

- Being bitten by a mosquito (*Safe*)

- Drinking alcohol (*Caution*) (*Note*: This is a risk because it decreases decision-making skills.)

- Sharing needles for ear piercing (*Stop*)

- Intercourse with a condom (*Caution*)

- Getting a blood transfusion after 1986 (*Safe*)

- Donating blood (*Safe*)

- Intercourse using only birth control pills (*Stop*)

- Oral sex without a condom or dental dam (*Stop*) (*Note*: explain dental dam or use of saran wrap.)

- Tattooing with unsterile equipment (*Stop*)

- Using an oil-based lubricant with a condom (*Stop*)

- Foreplay (*Caution*)

- Dry kissing (*Safe*)

- Masturbation (*Safe*)

- Cleaning an injection drug needle with water and then using it (*Stop*)

- Massage (*Safe*)

Notes for Group Leaders: You might need to describe anal intercourse. (When a man puts his penis into another person's rectum or asshole. The other person can be male or female.) You should explain that, because the anus is small and there is no lubrication, even when someone uses a condom this is still a risky behavior; however, a condom is better than no condom, and using a water-based lubricant can also lower the risk.

---

3 When you have read all the behaviors, ask the following questions:

- How is HIV transmitted from one person to another? (HIV is spread through the exchange of the body fluids of blood, semen, vaginal fluids or breastmilk. It can be spread by having unprotected intercourse—vaginal, oral or anal; by sharing needles; and from a mother to her unborn child.)

- How do we know that casual contact (hugging, holding hands, kissing) does not spread HIV? (HIV is only spread through the body fluids of blood, semen and vaginal fluids; it cannot be spread if there is not an exchange of these fluids.)

- If a risk is uncertain, how can a person decide about that behavior? (If you are uncertain about the risk of a behavior it is better to avoid it until you know. You can call 1-800-432-AIDS to get more information. We will talk more about getting information in the next session.)

- How can you prevent HIV transmission? (The best way to protect yourself is not to have sex or use drugs, especially drugs where you are sharing needles. If you do have sex, you should always use a latex condom.)

4 During the discussion, brainstorm a list of safe and safer sex guidelines for teens. Remember to emphasize the broad nature of sexuality and caring about another person. Examples of risk-free activities include talking, touching, massaging and dancing. Low-risk activities include vaginal intercourse with a latex condom and French kissing.

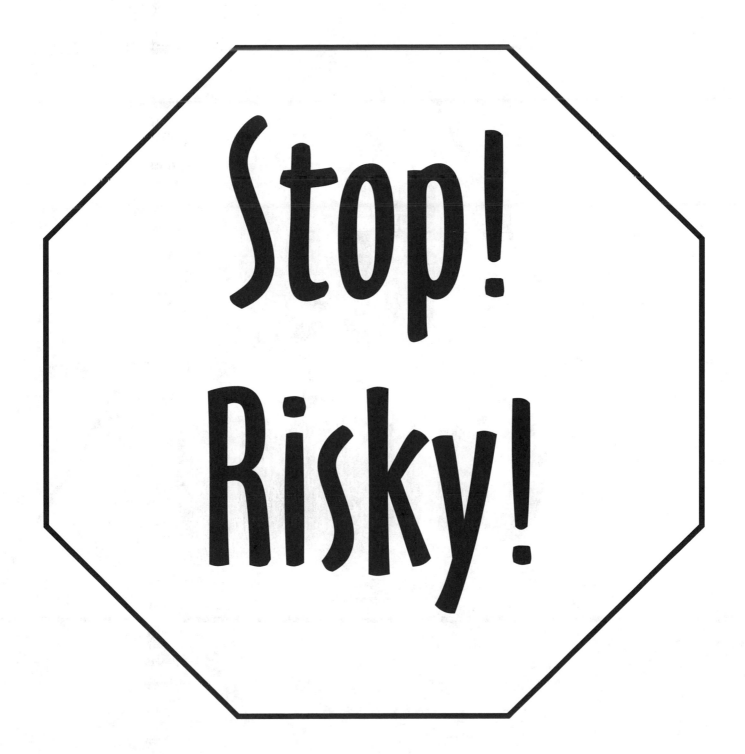

Sample Sign

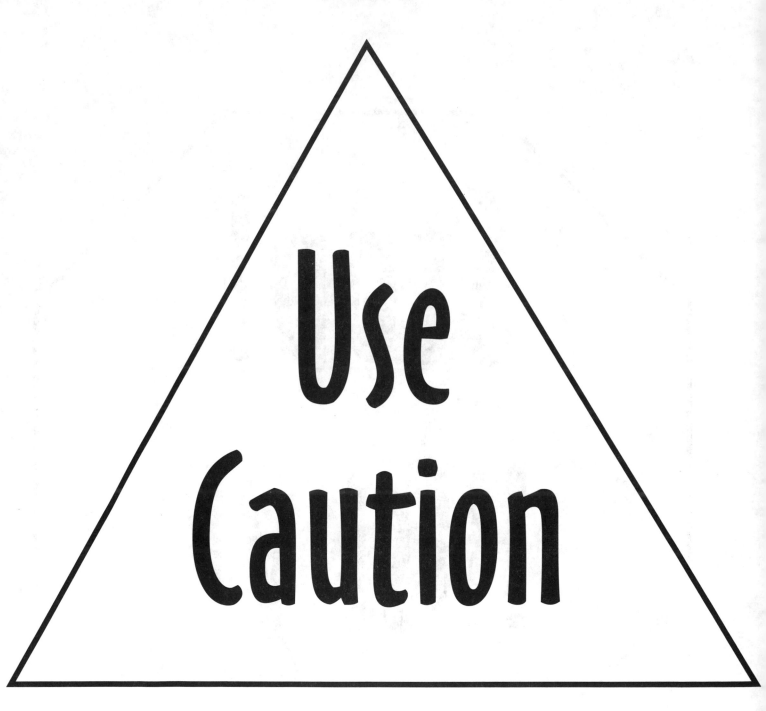

Sample Sign

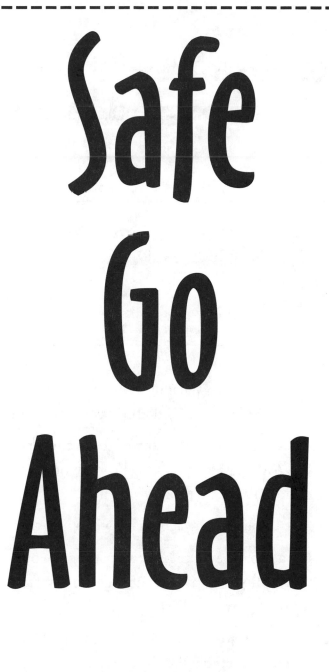

3.

What Are You Concerned About?

☺ **Objective:**   Youth will identify areas of personal concern and learn that some of their concerns are shared by others.

🕐 **Time:**   10 minutes

✂ **Materials:**   Newsprint and markers

Procedure

1 Ask the group: What are some things in your life that you are concerned about? Write their concerns on newsprint.

If they don't bring up any of these concerns, suggest the following: HIV/AIDS, people their age (or anyone) selling drugs, people having children at a young age, violence.

2 Ask: What feelings come up when you think about this concern?

On a separate piece of newsprint, list words that reflect the feelings raised. If youth have trouble getting started, ask if they feel any of the following: worried? scared? sad?

3 Ask youth to identify the concerns and feelings that seem to be shared by many members of the group.

4 Summarize by letting youth know that these concerns and feelings are normal. Let them know that during the sessions that follow they will learn methods to help them stay safer and reduce their fears.

Notes for Group Leaders: Save the newsprint lists to use later.

4.

Why Do People Feel Invulnerable?

☺ **Objective:**	Youth will understand reasons teens often feel invulnerable and how this may increase their risk taking.
⏰ **Time:**	10 minutes
✂ **Materials:**	None

Procedure

1 Define "invulnerable." (Feeling like nothing bad can happen to you; invincible.)

2 Lead a discussion using the following questions.

For all youth:

- Do most people your age who sell drugs think they might get caught? Why or why not?

- Do people your age who are having sex worry about getting an STD? Why or why not?

- What do people your age think will happen to them if they hook (cut, skip) school?

- What do people your age think will happen if they carry weapons? if they play with guns?

- Do people your age think they will get pregnant or get someone pregnant if they have sex? Why or why not?

- How might alcohol and other drugs make you feel invulnerable? What can you do about this?

- Are there certain groups of people who are at risk for HIV or drug use?

Explain that there is no such thing as a "risk group"—only risky behaviors. Ask: If you have learned that someone you know has HIV or AIDS, did you find yourself looking for ways you are different from this person and therefore won't get HIV yourself? Have group members give examples.

For older youth only:

- Has anyone had the experience of feeling invulnerable one night, but feeling regretful or scared the next morning?

- How does being "turned on" or feeling horny (sexually aroused), make you feel safe (as though the person must be OK)? Is there any similarity between the effects of drugs and the effect of sexual arousal on judgment?

- Does being "in love" or being with a partner for a long time make us feel safe and invulnerable with that person? Is this a reasonable way to feel? What is a long time? What can we do to prevent false feelings of safety in ourselves or in others?

- Does carrying a condom make you feel as if you are preparing to have sex? Is it wrong for a girl to plan on having sex? How can these feelings put someone at risk?

3 Summarize by letting youth know that many times people their age feel invulnerable and therefore put themselves at increased risk. It is important that they think about a behavior and what kind of risk it might put them in before they do it.

5.

Defining a Value

☺ **Objective:** Youth will develop an understanding of the term "value."

🕑 **Time:** 5 minutes

✂ **Materials:** Newsprint and markers

Procedure

1 Explain that a value is a strongly held belief. Write the definition on newsprint. Give examples of personal values such as: "Education is important," "Sex is something that should be thought about seriously," "Family is important."

2 Ask youth to give some examples of values.

3 Briefly discuss where values come from. (*Example:* family, friends, TV, school, church, etc.)

4 Emphasize that values are personal. Each person's job is to decide on his or her own personal values. Values help determine the choices we make and the way we behave.

Notes for Group Leaders: This session may be quite variable in length and intensity, but generally will be short. Once you have explained what "values" are, don't push the discussion if youth are not interested. Instead move quickly to the next activity (Rank Your Values).

6.

Rank Your Values

Source: Planned Parenthood of Maryland's STARS (Students Talking About Responsible Sexuality).

☺ **Objective:** Youth will identify and rank some of their personal values.

🕐 **Time:** 20 minutes

✂ **Materials:** **Rank Your Values** worksheet, 1 for each participant

Scissors

Clear tape

Pieces of colored 8-1/2" x 11" paper

Procedure

1 Distribute the **Rank Your Values** worksheet. Have youth cut the worksheet into strips. Give each youth a blank sheet of colored paper to sort their values on. Tell youth that one way to find out what your values are is to rank them—selecting the one that is most important, the one that is second-most important, and so on.

Give each participant a table or floor space, large enough to lay out all of the value statements. The group leaders should also participate.

2 Tell youth to look over the value statements carefully and to move them around until they have a list with their most important value at the top and their least important value at the bottom.

Caution them to work slowly and think carefully about each statement. They may change the order of the statements if they change their minds—the ranking should show how they really feel about the statements. They should tape the statements in their final order to the piece of colored paper. Allow time to work.

3 Remind youth of groundrules. Then go around the room and have each youth share (if willing) her or his most important item, second item, third item, second to last item, least important item, etc. The group leaders should also share.

4 After everyone has had an opportunity to share, lead a discussion using the following questions:

- What might be the reason for the different values in the group? (different families, religions, genders, ages, etc.)

- If the group leaders' ranking differs a lot from the rest of the group, why might that be? (older, different culture, etc.)

- How would your family rank the items?

- Can you think of any important values that aren't listed here?

5 Summarize by stating that we all need to think about our values and what is most important to us when we make decisions and when we decide how we will behave.

Notes for Group Leaders: Have several rolls of tape for youth to use. Running a long piece of tape over each participant's value strips is an easy way to hold the strips in place.

Worksheet

Rank Your Values

Cut the statements into strips along the lines.
Then put them in order from most important to least important to you.

Making it on my own

Getting good grades

Preparing for my future

Getting along with my parents

Getting married

Living by my religion

Being artistic or creative

Making money

Being popular with my friends

Getting a job I really like

Being good in sports

Having children

Making new friends

Having my own car

7.

Values Voting

Source: Planned Parenthood of Maryland's STARS (Students Talking About Responsible Sexuality).

☺	**Objective:**	Youth will identify personal values about relationships and sexuality and discuss them with other youth.
⏱	**Time:**	20–60 minutes (depending on how many items are read and discussed)
✂	**Materials:**	"Agree" and "Disagree" signs (See samples on page 70 and 71.)
		List of **Values Voting Items,** for group leaders (See page 69.)

Procedure

1 Remind youth of the groundrules established in Session 1:

- Respect each other. Don't talk out of turn.

- Keep confidentiality. Don't discuss what is said outside of the group.

- Everyone has a right to his or her opinion.

2 Put the "Agree" and "Disagree" signs at opposite ends of the room.

3 Explain that you will be reading a statement and youth are to decide whether they agree or disagree with the statement. Without following their friends, they should move to the side of the room that reflects their own personal decision. (*Note:* Encourage youth to pick a side for each item; they may stand in the middle if they cannot decide.)

4 Read each statement on the **Values Voting Items** page and encourage youth to move quickly to the Agree or Disagree sides of the room.

5 For each item, ask 1 person from each side to offer his or her reason for choosing that side. Encourage others to speak if they like. This exercise may emphasize differences and it is important that all group members understand that differences are expected and accepted.

6 When all statements have been read, have youth return to their seats.

7 Lead a discussion using the following questions:

- What made it easy to pick a side?

- What made it hard to pick a side?

- Why did people want to stand in the middle?

- Did this activity make you think about things you usually take for granted?

- How would your parents have chosen?

- Share 1 area where you and your parents might have different feelings.

- Were there any items you think that boys and girls would have different feelings about?

8 Summarize by asking what youth learned about their values from this activity. Help them identify how understanding their values might help them make decisions (e.g., it is easier to carry out a decision that is supported by your values).

Notes for Group Leaders: Play "devil's advocate" to make sure a range of views are given. It is important for the group leaders to support youth in minority positions for having the courage to have a different opinion. Sometimes this can be done simply by standing next to them on the minority side.

Make sure you remain objective. The goal is to help youth clarify their values, not convince them of yours. Help youth to be tolerant of differences and make sure that they listen to different points of view—they might change their minds when they listen to others' reasons.

Youth usually learn from and enjoy this game a lot. If time is limited, just read half of the items so you have enough time for discussion.

Group Leader

Values Voting Items

1. Men should be able to cry.

2. Teens should be able to get birth control without their parents' consent.

3. If a woman is pregnant and HIV positive, she should get an abortion.

4. Condoms should be given out free of charge to anyone who wants them.

5. I would approve of an interracial relationship for myself.

6. When a girl says No to sex, a guy should believe her.

7. By wearing tight clothing a women is saying she wants to have sex.

8. It's important to make a lot of money.

9. Gay people should be able to adopt children.

10. It should be against the law for people with HIV to have sex.

Agree

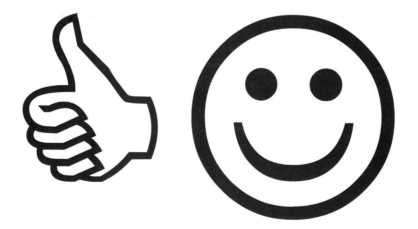

Disagree

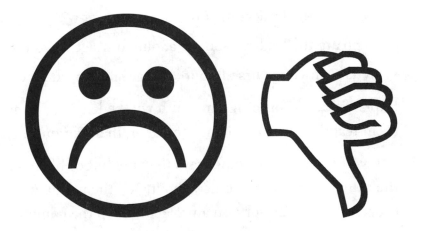

8. ✓ **What Youth Can Do**

☺ **Objective:**   Youth learn that they can take responsibility for their concerns.

🕐 **Time:**   10 minutes

✂ **Materials:**   Newsprint with list from What Are You Concerned About? activity.

Procedure

1 Refer to the concerns list generated at the beginning of the session and invite youth to think back on what they said they were concerned about. Ask:

- Which historical leaders have changed peoples' concerns in the past?

- Has anyone from your community changed peoples' concerns?

- Who are the leaders in your community now?

- Who are the leaders who are about your age in your community?

- What can you yourself do to change some of these concerns?

2 Explain that in this program youth will be learning things to help them teach others and change things in their community.

3 Ask youth to suggest some ways they might be able to change some of the things they are concerned about. Tell them that at the end of the program they will work on a project to help the community.

Notes for Group Leaders: This discussion can bring up many situations that youth cannot do much to change (e.g., family or friends with serious drug addictions, police violence). Help youth focus on the individual choices they can make for themselves. Also have them focus on their friends who have not become involved in drugs (either selling or using) or sex. Ask how youth can help prevent these people from starting.

---

9. Wrap-Up and Closing Ritual

☺ **Objective:**	Youth will provide feedback on Session 2 and summarize what they have learned.
🕐 **Time:**	5 minutes
✂ **Materials:**	None

Procedure

1 Have the group sit in a circle. Perform the chosen closing ritual.

2 Gather feedback about the day's session by asking the following questions:

- What did they like?

- What didn't they like?

- What did they learn?

- What would they like to learn more about at another session?

3 Remind the youth of the next meeting time and place. Tell them to remind each other. Offer to give them a call the night before the meeting.

4 Provide a way for youth to contact you if they need to and remind them that they can use the Question Box.

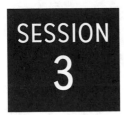

Educate Yourself: Obtaining Information

Purpose	Youth will learn ways to obtain information in order to make good decisions.

Session Overview
(100 minutes)

1 Opening Ritual and Review (10 minutes)

2 SODA Decision-Making Model: Step 2 (10 minutes)

3 Finding Information for Good Decisions (10 minutes)

4 Telephone Exercise: Gathering Information (25 minutes)

5 Video: What Kids Want to Know About Sex and Growing Up (35 minutes)

6 Field Assignments (5 minutes)

7 Wrap-Up and Closing Ritual (5 minutes)

Preparation

Pre-Session Activities

❏ Read over and become familiar with Session 3 activities.

❏ Prepare snacks.

❏ Prepare a "Resource Guide for Youth." It should include various places for youth to get information or counseling. Look in your local phone book or call your local health department to find potential resources.

Good resources to include are topic-specific hotlines, crisis lines, local health department, social workers, counselors, teen clinics, family planning clinics, sexual assault centers, churches and a general youth hotline. Include the listings from **National Resources for Youth,** page 90.

❏ Prepare Field Assignments chart. This can show how many field assignments each youth has completed. If possible, it helps to provide incentives for youth to complete field assignments, e.g., if they complete 3 assignments they get free movie passes. (See Sample on page 97.)

Materials

❏ snacks

❏ Family Tree, Groundrules, SODA Model and Field Assignments charts

❏ masking tape

❏ pencils

❏ copies of field assignment worksheets **Condom Hunt** and **Parent Interview** (See pages 95 and 96.)

❏ newsprint

❏ markers

❏ *Resource Guide for Youth*, 1 for each participant

❏ telephone

❏ telephone book

❏ video: *What Kids Want to Know about Sex and Growing Up* (Available from ETR Associates: 1-800-321-4407.)

❏ TV and VCR

I. Opening Ritual and Review

☺ **Objective:**	Youth will review highlights from Session 2.
⏱ **Time:**	10 minutes
✂ **Materials:**	None

Procedure

I After the opening ritual, sit down with youth and remind them of groundrules.

2 Answer any questions from the Question Box.

3 Review Session 2 by asking the following questions:

- What is a value?

- What does "invulnerable" mean?

- In what ways does alcohol make you feel invulnerable?

- What are some other reasons youth may feel invulnerable?

- What is one way you can change some of the concerns we identified in the last session?

2.

SODA Decision-Making Model—Step 2: Options

Source: S. Schinke, A. Gordon and R. Weston. 1990. Self-Instruction to Prevent HIV Infection Among African-American and Hispanic-American Adolescents. Journal of Consulting and Clinical Psychology 58 (4): 432-436.

☺ **Objective:** Youth will learn decision making, with a focus on Step 2: Options.

🕐 **Time:** 10 minutes

✂ **Materials:** SODA Model chart, newsprint and markers

Procedure

I Briefly review the first step of decision making.

Step I: Stop—**Stop and state the problem.** Pause and give yourself time to decide what the problem really is.

2 Explain that today's lesson will concentrate on the next step of decision making—Options.

Step 2: Options—**Consider the options** or choices and the consequences of those choices. Educate yourself so you know all the choices and consequences before you make a decision.

3 Read 2 of the following vignettes and have youth brainstorm a list of information needed to make an informed decision for each situation. Write the list on newsprint.

For younger youth:

You have the chance to go to a different elementary school/middle school. At the new school, they have special programs that are interesting. But you would have to switch schools in the middle of the year.

* What is the problem? *(to switch schools or stay were you are)*

* How would you be feeling? *(Possible answers: scared, excited, uncertain)*

- What do you need to know about before you make your decision? *(Possible answers: How far away is the school? Are there other schools that have similar programs? What are the special programs like? What are the students like? What classes could you take? What do this school's graduates do? etc.)*

- What are your options? *(Possible answers: switch schools; remain at your school; switch schools at a later date; etc.)*

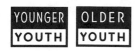

For younger and older boys:

Tavon and his girlfriend have been going together for 2 months. Tavon has never had sex before. He has heard from his friends that his girlfriend has had several boyfriends before. He assumes that she will start wanting to have sex soon. All his friends have been bugging him and asking him if they are having sex.

One day they get out of school early, and Tavon's girlfriend invites him over to her house to watch TV. Tavon wants his friend, Larry, to come with them but his girlfriend says Larry gets on her nerves and she wants it to be just them. Tavon is a little worried about going because he knows his girlfriend's mother is never home during the day and they will be all alone.

- What is the problem? *(whether or not to go to his girlfriend's house, whether or not to have sex)*

- How does Tavon feel? How does his girlfriend feel?
  (Possible answers: scared, excited, upset, nervous)

- What does Tavon need to know before he makes his decision?
  (Possible answers: What are the consequences of having sex? of not having sex? How can he tell his girlfriend he isn't ready? What kind of protection would he need if he was ready?)

- What are Tavon's options?
  (Possible answers: Go to her house but make sure they don't have sex; tell her he's busy; invite Larry anyway; suggest alternate activities—rec center, movie, the park, a friend's house.)

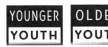

For younger and older girls:

Chantel and her boyfriend have been going together for 2 months. Chantel has never had sex before. She has heard from her friends that her boyfriend has had several girlfriends before. She assumes that he will start wanting to have sex soon.

One day they get out of school early, and Chantel's boyfriend invites her over to his house to watch TV. Chantel wants her friend, Latrice, to come with them but her boyfriend says Latrice gets on his nerves and he wants it to be just them. Chantel is a little worried about going because she knows her boyfriend's mother is never home during the day and they will be all alone.

- What is the problem? *(whether or not to go to her boyfriend's house, whether or not to have sex)*

- How does Chantel feel? How does her boyfriend feel? *(Possible answers: scared, excited, upset, nervous)*

- What does Chantel need to know before she makes her decision? *(Possible answers: What are the consequences of having sex? of not having sex? How can she tell her boyfriend she isn't ready? What kind of protection would she need if she was ready?)*

- What are Chantel's options? *(Possible answers: Go to his house but make sure they don't have sex; tell him she's busy; invite Latrice anyway; suggest alternate activities— rec center, movie, the park, a friend's house.)*

For older boys only:

Remember Tavon? He has been going with his girlfriend for over a year. They are both in love. They started having sex about a month ago and up to this point Tavon has always used a condom. She is beginning to complain about it now. She says it takes the feeling away and she doesn't want to use one anymore.

- What is the problem? *(whether or not to keep using condoms)*

- How does each of them feel?
  (*Possible answers: scared, angry, hurt, sad, frustrated*)

- What information will Tavon need to know to make this decision?
  (*Possible answers: What are the consequences of having sex without protection? of not having sex? What kind of protection does he need? Where can he get condoms? How can he find out more about HIV/STD? How can he explain to his girlfriend the importance of using condoms without offending her?*)

- What are Tavon's options?
  (*Possible answers: Break up with his girlfriend; say it's condoms or no sex; give in to her request; have her go with him to a clinic to get tested for HIV and other STD, and get birth control.*)

For older girls only:

Remember Chantel? She has been going with her boyfriend for over a year. They are both in love. They started having sex about a month ago and up to this point her boyfriend has always used a condom. He is beginning to complain about it now. He says it takes the feeling away and he doesn't want to use one anymore.

- What is the problem? (*whether or not to keep using condoms*)

- How does each of them feel?
  (*Possible answers: scared, angry, hurt, sad, frustrated*)

- What does Chantel need to know before she makes her decision?
  (*Possible answers: What are the consequences of having sex without protection? of not having sex? What kind of protection does she need? Where can she get condoms? How can she find out more about HIV/STD? How can she explain to her boyfriend the importance of using condoms without offending him?*)

- What are Chantel's options?
  (*Possible answers: Break up with her boyfriend; say it's condoms or no sex; give in to his request; have him go with her to a clinic to get tested for HIV and other STD, and get birth control.*)

4 Explain to youth that next week they will look at Step 3: Decide. To decide, they must compare the good and bad things about the options. But before they are able to decide they need to learn how to gather information about each of the options. In the next activity, they will learn different methods to gather information and explore the positive and negative things about each option.

Notes for Group Leaders: Ask youth to be specific. For example, when discussing "Don't have sex," be sure to help youth identify other options, such as finding fun ways to be together that don't involve sex, or finding different ways to please a partner without sex (e.g., kissing, rubbing, mutual masturbation). If "Explain the dangers of not using a condom" is given as an option, get youth to identify what those dangers are.

You may need to adapt the vignettes for your target audience. Use characters from the Family Tree in Session 1. Younger youth may have difficulty discussing the sexual activity vignettes. Try and give them prompts but if the conversation is not moving at all, don't persist for more than a couple of minutes.

---

3. Finding Information for Good Decisions

☺ **Objective:**	Youth will identify potential resources to learn about options.	
	Youth will learn how to gather information about options and resources.	
🕐 **Time:**	10 minutes	
✂ **Materials:**	Newsprint and markers	
	Resource Guide for Youth	

Procedure

1 Review the list of information that youth said they would need to make a decision from the SODA Step 2: Options activity. Have them brainstorm how and where they might get the information for each situation. List their suggestions on newsprint. If they have trouble, help them with the examples provided (see page 86). There are several additional vignettes to explore (see page 87) if time permits.

2 As you review the lists, discuss the strengths and weaknesses of each information source by asking the following questions.

- Why might this be a good source? Why not?

- What different information might you get from each source?

Explain that each source can provide different kinds of information, and that they may have to get information from several different sources to make a well-informed decision.

3 Ask youth how they would locate each source to get the information they needed. *Examples:*

- Where would they get the number of the clinic?

- How would they get an appointment with their teacher?

> • How can they set up a time to talk with the counselor?

Encourage youth to use the actual words they would say. For example, instead of saying, "I would talk to a counselor" ask them to say *exactly* what they would say.

4 Provide guidelines for talking to an adult:

> • Try to relax.
>
> • Write down what you want to say ahead of time.
>
> • Find a good time for both you and the adult.
>
> • Start with a direct statement: I want to talk about something private that is very important to me.

5 Pass out the *Resource Guide for Youth*.

Notes for Group Leaders: If youth begin to get restless, move along quickly. If youth are looking bored, discuss only 1 vignette.

Examples for Vignettes from Activity 2

YOUNGER YOUTH **For younger youth:**

Where would you get the information about whether or not to change schools?

What information do you need?	**Where do you get information?**
What do most students do after they graduate?	Talk to principal
What kind of programs do they have?	Talk to other students
What are the students like?	Talk to teachers
What are the teachers like?	Talk to former graduates
Are there any extra costs?	Talk to counselors from the school
	Spend a day at the school

YOUNGER YOUTH **OLDER YOUTH** **For younger and older boys/girls:**

Where would Chantel/Tavon get the information to help her/him
make a decision about whether or not to have sex?

What information do you need?	**Where do you get information?**
What are the consequences?	Talk to parents, relatives or other adults
How good are condoms at protecting you?	Talk to close friends
How do you use a condom?	Talk to boyfriend/girlfriend about the decision
Where can you get condoms?	Go to a clinic
How can you tell a partner if you're not interested in having sex?	Talk to a doctor or nurse
	Call the AIDS hotline or a teen hotline
	Go to a drug store
	Go to the health department
	Read a brochure
	Get a book from the library on growing up and sex

Optional Vignettes

(Use if time allows.)

1. If a friend came to you and thought he/she had a sexually transmitted disease, what kind of information would you try and help your friend find and how might he/she get it?

What information do you need?

Information on HIV/STD testing

Information about how to use a condom

Help on how to tell partners they might be infected

Information on AIDS and HIV infection

Symptoms of STD

Where do you get information?

Call a clinic

Read a book from the library

Ask a teacher

Look at pamphlets from a clinic or school

Talk to an older sister/brother

2. If a friend came to you and thought she was pregnant or he had gotten someone pregnant, what kind of information would you try and help your friend find and where might she/he find it?

What information do you need?

Information on pregnancy testing

Information on prenatal care

Information on adoption

Information on abortion

Information on HIV/STD

Information on birth control

Information on programs/schools for pregnant teens

Where do you get information?

Parents

Clinic or health department

Library

Counselor

Older adult

Teacher

4.

Telephone Exercise: Gathering Information

☺ **Objective:**   Youth will practice gathering information from different sources.

🕐 **Time:**   25 minutes

✂ **Materials:**   Telephone, telephone book

Resource Guide for Youth

Procedure

1 Explain to youth that they are now going to practice obtaining different types of information for decision making.

Ask youth where they could get information about symptoms of STD. If they mention a clinic or doctor, ask them how they would get the number.

Have a volunteer call Information to get the number of a clinic. Have another volunteer call the clinic and obtain information about their services and how to make an appointment.

2 Have several youth take turns calling the National AIDS Hotline, 1-800-342-AIDS, and asking a question about HIV or AIDS. If they are comfortable, have youth report back to the group. (*Note:* You may want to brainstorm several questions before the volunteers call.)

3 Have youth look up the number for the local health department or Planned Parenthood in the phone book. Have them call to ask what services the agency offers.

4 Pass out the *Resource Guide for Youth.* Have a volunteer call one of the hotlines or services listed and ask a question.

Have this youth report back on the call.

Notes for Group Leaders: Remind youth to check to see if there is a charge to call Information (411) in their area. Make sure they understand the difference between 411 (Information), 311 (in some areas, police, non-emergency) and 911 (emergency number).

Tell them that they do not have to answer any questions that people on the hotline might ask them. They can say, "I do not want to answer that question."

Group Leader

National Resources
for Youth

National Sexual Assault Hotline: 1-800-656-HOPE (4673)

National AIDS Clearinghouse: 1-800-458-5231

National AIDS Hotline: 1-800-342-AIDS (2437);
  (in Spanish) 1-800-344-7432

Childhelp East: 1-800-422-4453 (A national 24-hour crisis intervention
  hotline for child/adult abuse and family violence)

Child Find of America, Inc.: 1-800-426-5678 (Runaways)

National Youth Crisis Hotline: 1-800-442-4673

National Clearinghouse for Alcohol and Drug Information:
  1-800-729-6686

The Center for Substance Abuse Treatment Hotline:
  1-800-662-HELP (4357) (24 hours)

National Job Corps: 1-800-733-5627

STD Hotline: 1-800-227-8922 (8 a.m.-11 p.m.)

5.

Video: What Kids Want to Know About Sex and Growing Up

☺ **Objective:**   Youth will learn accurate information about puberty.

🕐 **Time:**   35 minutes

✂ **Materials:**   TV and VCR

What Kids Want to Know About Sex and Growing Up video (Available from ETR Associates, 1-800-321-4407)

Procedure

1   Explain that youth are going to watch a video about puberty and growing up that will provide lots of information that will help them make decisions as they face different issues and challenges during adolescence. Tell them they can share what they learn with their parents. Explain that a family's personal values and beliefs play a large role in how children think about sex and that it is important for them to talk to their parents about this issue.

Show youth the first 30 minutes of the video *What Kids Want to Know about Sex and Growing Up.* (*Note:* Stop the video when it reaches the parent section.)

2   Lead a discussion about the information presented in the video using the following questions:

- What changes happen to girls during puberty?
  - *Body sweats more.*
  - *Skin and hair become more oily.*
  - *Body has sudden growth spurt.*
  - *Soft, darker hair grows around the vulva and later becomes curly, thick and coarse.*

>   *– Hair grows under the arms.*
>
>   *– Breasts and nipples gradually grow larger and fuller.*
>
>   *– Nipples may become a darker color.*
>
>   *– Menstrual periods begin.*

- Is there a normal age when girls should get their period? (*No, there is a large range of ages that are normal.*)

- What changes happen to boys during puberty?

  – Testicles gradually grow larger and fuller.

  – Penis gradually grows larger and longer.

  – Body sweats more.

  – Skin and hair become more oily.

  – Soft, darker hair grows around the base of the penis and later becomes curly, thick and coarse.

  – Hair grows under the arms.

  – Hair grows on the face, first the mustache then the beard and sideburns.

  – Hair may grow on chest.

  – The voice cracks and then becomes deeper.

  – Sperm begin to be produced.

  – Ejaculations—including wet dreams—begin to occur.

- Is there a normal age when boys should get facial hair? (*No, there is a large range of ages that are normal.*)

- Why do some kids feel uncomfortable with the changes happening to their bodies?

3 Summarize that it is important to gain information about puberty to understand themselves better. Stress that the more information we have, the more we are able to make good decisions.

Field Assignments

6.

☺ **Objective:**	Youth will get practice gathering information and resources from different sources.
⏱ **Time:**	5 minutes
✂ **Materials:**	Field Assignment worksheets: **Condom Hunt** and **Parent Interview**
	Field Assignment chart (See sample, page 97.)

Procedure

I Explain that for the rest of the program, youth can choose 1 field assignment to do each week. Explain that there will be time for each person to share the outcome of her or his assignment. If possible, offer incentives such as fast food gift certificates, ball game passes, etc. Document how many assignments each youth has completed on the Field Assignment chart.

2 Review the possible field assignments and have youth select which they want to do. Distribute worksheets as needed.

Field assignments:

- Call the National AIDS Hotline and ask a question you have about HIV or AIDS (1-800-432-AIDS).

- Go on a condom hunt. (See **Condom Hunt** worksheet for specific instructions.)

- Interview different parents about their daily tasks. You must interview at least 2 different types of parents: a teen parent and an older parent, a parent of young children and a parent whose children are grown, etc. (See **Parent Interview** worksheet for specific instructions.)

- Call 1 of the numbers on the *Resource Guide for Youth* and ask what services the agency provides. Report back to the group.

Notes for Group Leaders: You can add more field assignments depending on the interest of the group members.

Probably only a few youth will do this activity each week, but try and encourage the others by supporting those youth who complete the assignments.

Name _____

Condom Hunt

Name of store: _____   Store hours: _____

1. Are there any signs in the store to identify birth control or family planning items?

   ❏ Yes   ❏ No

2. Are all the family planning methods in the same place?   ❏ Yes   ❏ No

3. Did you talk to any of the store employees?   ❏ Yes   ❏ No
   (For example, ask: "Can you please tell me where the condoms are?")

   If yes, how did they react?   ❏ Positive ☺   ❏ Negative ☹   ❏ Neutral 😐

4. Where are the condoms located?

   ❏ Behind a counter   ❏ Next to a counter

   ❏ With the feminine hygiene products   ❏ Family planning section   ❏ Other

5. What is the cheapest price for 3 condoms? _____

6. Does the store have the following kinds of condoms?

Lubricated	❏ Yes	❏ No	❏ Don't know
Non-lubricated	❏ Yes	❏ No	❏ Don't know
With spermicide	❏ Yes	❏ No	❏ Don't know

7. Does the store have the following kinds of family planning methods?

Foam/Jelly	❏ Yes	❏ No	❏ Don't know
Spermicides	❏ Yes	❏ No	❏ Don't know

8. Where are these other family planning methods located?

   ❏ Behind a counter   ❏ Next to a counter

   ❏ With the feminine hygiene products   ❏ Family planning section   ❏ Other

Source: Adapted from Center for Population Options' Guide to Implementing TAP (Teens for AIDS Prevention Peer Education Program).

Worksheet

Name _____

Parent Interview

Interview at least 2 parents from different families. Interview different types of parents: grandparents raising children, married or single parents, older or younger parents, etc.

Find out the positive and negative changes having a baby had on their lives in these areas:

1. Friends and social life _____

   _____

2. Family relationships _____

   _____

3. Education and career plans _____

   _____

4. Money and finances _____

   _____

5. Daily routine and free time _____

   _____

Some rules for interviewing:

1. Explain what you are doing and how long the interview will take.

2. If someone does not want to answer a question, don't push it. Go on to another question.

3. Try to write down notes about what you think was most interesting.

4. Thank the person after the interview.

Source: Planned Parenthood of Maryland's STARS (Students Talking About Responsible Sexuality).

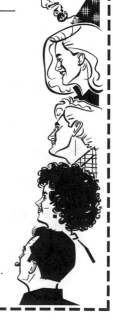

Sample Chart

Field Assignments

Name	Condom Hunt	Parent Interview	Talk w/ Parent	Calls to Hotline, etc.	Other

7. Wrap-Up and Closing Ritual

☺ **Objective:**	Youth will provide feedback on Session 3 and summarize what they have learned.
🕐 **Time:**	5 minutes
✂ **Materials:**	None

Procedure

1 Have group sit in a circle. Perform the chosen closing ritual.

2 Gather feedback about the day's session by asking the following questions:

- What did they like?

- What didn't they like?

- What did they learn?

- What would they like to learn more about at another session?

3 Remind youth of the next meeting time and place. Tell them to remind each other. Offer to give them a call the night before the meeting.

4 Provide a way for youth to contact you if they need to and remind them that they can use the Question Box.

Educate Yourself: Examining Consequences

Purpose	Youth will learn to weigh the positive and negative consequences of options as they make decisions.

Session Overview
(85 minutes)

1 **Opening Ritual and Review** (15 minutes)

2 **Parent Roleplay** (15–20 minutes)

3 **M&M's Game: How Many Kids Are Really...?** (15 minutes)

4 **Condom Demonstration** (10 minutes)

5 **Condom Race** (10 minutes)

6 **SODA Decision-Making Model: Step 3** (15 minutes)

7 **Wrap-Up and Closing Ritual** (5 minutes)

Preparation

Pre-Session Activities

❑ Read over and become familiar with Session 4 activities.

❑ Prepare snacks.

❑ *Optional:* Prepare permission slips for all-day retreat. Consult with your agency to determine the type of permission and legal releases you need to transport youth.

Materials

❑ snacks

❑ Family Tree, Groundrules, SODA Model and Field Assignment charts

❑ masking tape

❑ field assignment worksheets from Session 3

❑ newsprint

❑ markers

❑ props for Parent Roleplay (scarves, baseball cap)

❑ M&M's candies (approximately 100 pieces)

❑ condoms (at least 2 for each participant)

❑ cucumbers or dildos

❑ petroleum jelly

❑ funnel

❑ container of water

❑ tub to hold the water when the condom bursts

❑ paper towels

❑ water-based lubricant (e.g., KY Jelly™)

❑ *Optional:* Permission slips for all-day retreat

I. Opening Ritual and Review

☺ **Objective:**	Youth will review highlights from Session 3.
⏱ **Time:**	15 minutes
✂ **Materials:**	None

Procedure

1 After the opening ritual, sit down with youth and remind them of groundrules.

2 Answer any questions from the Question Box.

3 Review Session 3 by asking the following questions:

- If you had a question about HIV or an STD, how would you find the answers? (Be specific—if you would go to a clinic, how would you choose the clinic, get an appointment, etc.)

- How do you decide whether or not someone is a good source of information?

- At what age do young people usually go through puberty?

4 Ask if any youth completed field assignments. Have volunteers share what they did and what they learned from their assignments.

2. **Parent Roleplay**

☺ **Objective:**   Youth will identify parents as potential resources.

🕐 **Time:**   15–20 minutes

✂ **Materials:**   Props, such as a scarf for the mother or grandmother or a baseball cap
for the father

Procedure

1 Begin with the group leaders modeling a short roleplay showing both a
negative parent-child discussion (e.g., the parent can be coming home
from a bad day at work and the child wants to talk about a problem
with a boyfriend or girlfriend as soon as the parent comes in the door)
and a positive parent-child discussion (e.g., parent and child choose a
time to talk in advance, the child is prepared and the parent is
receptive).

2 Review guidelines for talking to adults from Session 3:

   • Try to relax.

   • Write down what you want to say ahead of time.

   • Find a good time for both of you.

   • Start with a direct statement: "I want to talk about something
      private that is very important to me."

3 Have youth form pairs and do a roleplay about Tavon or Chantel (or
characters from your family tree version) talking to one of the adults
in the family about a problem (the problem may be thinking about
having sex, a partner is pressuring them, or a problem in school). Tell
them to use the guidelines for talking to adults when doing the

roleplays. Suggest they use the props to become the person they are playing. (Adults could include David, Mary, Esther, or a character from your adapted version.)

4 Discuss the positive and negative aspects of each roleplay:

- What did Tavon/Chantel do in the roleplay that you admire?

- Are there other things he/she could have done to make the conversation go easier?

- What did the adult do to help the conversation?

- How did Tavon/Chantel feel after talking to the parent?

- What did he/she gain from it?

5 Remind youth that some days are difficult for parents and sometimes they may say things they do not mean. Parents may also need time to think about what you have told them.

6 Ask the youth if there are any guidelines from their own experiences that they would like to add. Have them tell you how the guidelines might make communication with adults and parents better.

Notes for Group Leaders: Remember that parenting styles differ and youth might not think your roleplay is realistic or would work in their home. Help them find ways to talk to their parents in their own style.

3.

M&M's Game: How Many Kids Are Really...?

☺ **Objective:**	Youth will have a more realistic understanding of what HIV risks young people are taking.
⏱ **Time:**	15 minutes
✂ **Materials:**	100 M&M's candies
	2 sheets of paper

Procedure

1 Tell youth that lots of young people around their age in an East coast city were asked their thoughts about sex and HIV infection. They were also asked what things they were doing: Were they having sex? Did they use condoms? Did they sell drugs? etc. A computer was used to ask the questions and nobody's name was attached to the answers. Explain that today you will share some of the things these young people said.

2 Ask a volunteer to illustrate, using M&M's, how many kids their age out of 100 he or she thinks are having sex. Have the volunteer put the number of kids (M&M's) having sex on a sheet of paper. Ask the group if they think the volunteer's estimate is right.

- Show them, with M&M's, how many youth this age actually are having sex: 37%. (See Notes for Group Leaders on page 105.) Count out 37 M&M's by taking away or adding to the youth's original estimate.

If the volunteer and/or group overestimated, ask:

- Why might you think more kids are having sex than actually are?

- Why would youth say they are having sex if they are not?

Ask another volunteer to illustrate how many of the kids who are having sex are using condoms. Again, have the group assess the estimate.

Then show them with the M&M's how many youth actually use condoms: 64%. Count out 64 M&M's.

If they overestimated or underestimated, ask why they think they did.

3 Repeat the same procedure for how many youth are selling drugs (6%). Ask:

- Why might people think more kids are selling drugs?

- Does everyone carrying a beeper sell drugs?

- Why do youth like beepers?

- Do youth want to look like they are selling drugs? If yes, why?

4 Repeat the same procedure for how many youth are using drugs (6%). If they overestimated or underestimated, ask them why they think they did. Ask:

- Do people who sell drugs use them?

- Why are people who use drugs more at risk for HIV infection? (because of using needles, and also because all drugs—including alcohol—can hurt your decision-making ability).

Notes for Group Leaders: All percentages stated in this session reflect the actual behavior of 9 to 15 year olds in the Baltimore area. You will want to use the actual percent for kids in your community. Statistics are available from the Centers for Disease Control and Prevention (CDC) publication Youth Risk Behavior Surveillance—United States, 1997, *Morbidity and Mortality Weekly Report*, Vol. 47, No. SS-3, August 14, 1998; or from your local health department or university.

---

4. Condom Demonstration

☺ **Objective:** Youth will learn accurate information about condom use.

🕐 **Time:** 10 minutes

✂ **Materials:** Condoms, cucumber or dildo

Petroleum jelly, funnel, container of water, tub to hold the water when the condom bursts, paper towels, water-based lubricant (e.g., KY Jelly™)

Procedure

1 Demonstrate the correct way to use a condom using the following steps:

1. Buy or get latex condoms. (Be sure they are latex, not lambskin, because the pores of lambskin condoms are larger and it is possible for HIV to get through the pores.)

2. Check the expiration date on the back of the condom package.

3. Discuss safer sex with your partner before you are aroused.

4. Place the condom on the man's erect penis.

5. Squeeze the air out of the tip of the condom. Make sure there is a space between the end of the penis and the tip of the condom to collect the semen.

6. Unroll the condom over the penis all the way to the base of the penis. Continue to hold on to the tip while you roll the condom down.

7. After intercourse, hold on to the rim of the condom while removing the penis (so the condom does not stay inside the partner).

8. Throw the used condom away properly. (Wrap in toilet paper and throw away in a trash can. Do not flush it down the toilet.)

2 To demonstrate how strong condoms are, how large they can get and the effect of oil-based lubricants, have volunteers fill up a condom with water (up to a gallon or so) and put an oil-based lubricant on the condom (petroleum jelly). By the end of the session, the condom will have disintegrated.

Emphasize the need to use water-based lubricants such as KY Jelly™ and other lubricants found with condoms in the store. Saliva will also work. In addition, give examples of oil-based lubricants (baby oil, hand cream, Vaseline™, etc.) that they should avoid.

Notes for Group Leaders: The condom might need some "wiggling" before it breaks. You can also fill 2 condoms and put Vaseline™ on one and KY Jelly™ on the other to compare which one breaks.

---

5. Condom Race

☺ **Objective:**	Youth will practice the proper way to put on a condom.	
⏲ **Time:**	10 minutes	
✄ **Materials:**	2 cucumbers or dildos	
	A condom for everyone in the group (plus extras for group members to take home)	

Procedure

1 Divide youth into 2 teams and give everyone a condom.

2 Have the teams stand in 2 lines and give the first person in each line a dildo or cucumber. Each person on the team must put the condom on the dildo or cucumber and take it off.

3 During the race, each person must show the condom to the group leader to make sure it has been put on correctly before passing the dildo or cucumber to the next team member. If the condom is not put on correctly, the person must try again until it is correct. The team that finishes first wins.

Notes for Group Leaders: Everyone has fun with this game. Be sure to watch youth putting on the condom to ensure they are doing it properly.

Have extra condoms for youth who want some. (Be sure you have permission from your sponsoring agency.) Before giving out condoms discuss responsible use of condoms (they are not to be used as water balloons, etc.). Be sure to collect used condoms at the end of the activity.

6. SODA Decision-Making Model—Step 3: Decide

Source: S. Schinke, A. Gordon and R. Weston. 1990. Self-Instruction to Prevent HIV Infection Among African-American and Hispanic-American Adolescents. Journal of Consulting and Clinical Psychology 58 (4): 432-436.

☺ **Objective:** Youth will acquire skills for decision making, with a focus on Step 3: Decide.

🕐 **Time:** 15 minutes

✂ **Materials:** SODA Model chart, newsprint and markers

Procedure

1 Briefly review the first 2 steps of decision making.

Step 1: Stop—**Stop and state the problem.** Pause and give yourself time to decide what the problem really is.

Step 2: Options—**Consider the options** or choices and the consequences of those choices. Educate yourself so you know all the choices and consequences before you make a decision.

2 Explain that today they are going to work on the third step—**Decide.**

Step 3: Decide—**Decide and choose the best solution** from the options. What is best will vary depending on the problem and your values (strongly held beliefs). Making a decision is done by weighing the advantages and disadvantages of the options.

YOUNGER YOUTH

For younger youth:

3 Review the first decision discussed in earlier sessions: whether or not to change schools to one that had interesting special programs. Ask:

- What are the different options we identified in the last session? (Review the options identified in Session 3.)

- What might be the positives and negatives of each choice?

Help youth identify the options and the consequences (good and bad) for each option. Record answers on newsprint in a chart format (see below).

Options	Good things about this option	Bad things about this option
_____	_____	_____
_____	_____	_____
_____	_____	_____
_____	_____	_____

Lead a short discussion about making a final decision. Ask:

- How would a person's values affect this decision?

- Which option would you choose?

- Why?

For older and younger youth:

4 Remind youth that another decision from earlier sessions was whether or not Tavon/Chantel should have sex. (*Note:* This is the first example for older youth.) Ask:

- What are the different options we identified in the last session?

- What might be some of the consequences of the different choices?

Prepare another chart with responses.

Probe for a variety of *different* consequences. For example, if youth say, "Mom would be mad at me" or "Dad would be mad at me," say, "OK—one consequence is that your parents might be mad at you. What's a different consequence?" If youth say, "get an STD," "get HIV," etc., ask, "What about that is bad?" This gets youth to begin to think about variations in severity of STD.

Lead a discussion using the following questions:

- How would Tavon/Chantel's values affect the decision? (Make sure examples are given that support both choices—to have sex and not to have sex).

- What would you decide for Tavon/Chantel?

- Why?

For older youth only:

5 Ask youth to think about the other decision from earlier sessions. Tavon/Chantel was deciding what to do about a girlfriend/boyfriend not wanting to use condoms. Review the options identified in Session 3.

Write the options on newsprint using the chart format to identify the good and bad consequences of each option. Add the idea of short-term versus long-term consequences by having youth think of consequences for both now and later (see below).

Options	Good things about this option		Bad things about this option	
	Now	Later	Now	Later
_____	_____		_____	
_____	_____		_____	
_____	_____		_____	
_____	_____		_____	

Suggest that youth might weigh options by asking: If I did this, what would be the positive and negative things for myself and others? Now? Later?

Again, encourage the youth to expand on different consequences.

Lead a discussion using the following questions:

- How would Tavon/Chantel's values affect this decision?

- What would you decide for Tavon/Chantel?

- Why?

6 Summarize by telling the youth that the next couple of sessions will concentrate on the skills they will need to carry out these decisions. They will learn communication skills, negotiation skills and more about sexual health.

Notes for Group Leaders: Keep this discussion as fast paced as possible. Try to make it as interactive as possible by consistently asking youth to give responses, rather than lecturing.

---

7. Additional Field Assignments

☺ **Objective:**	Youth will get experience gathering information and resources from different places.
⏰ **Time:**	5 minutes
✂ **Materials:**	Field Assignment worksheets

Procedure

1 Review the procedure for field assignments. Tell youth you are adding a couple of new assignments for them to chose from. Continue to provide the first 2 field assignment worksheets if youth want to do them. Remind youth that they must report what they have learned back to the group in order to receive any incentives being offered.

2 Give the following as an additional Field Assignment:

• Talk with a parent about what you have learned in the program and about what you can learn from her or him about decision making or gathering information.

Notes for Group Leaders: Probably only a few youth will do this activity each week but try and encourage other youth by supporting those who complete the assignments.

You can add more field assignments depending on the interest of the group members.

8.

Wrap-Up and Closing Ritual

☺ **Objective:**	Youth will provide feedback on Session 4 and summarize what they have learned.
🕐 **Time:**	5 minutes
✂ **Materials:**	None

Procedure

1 Have group sit in a circle. Perform the chosen closing ritual.

2 Gather feedback about the day's session by asking the following questions:

- What did they like?

- What didn't they like?

- What did they learn?

- What would they like to learn more about at another session?

3 Remind youth of the next meeting time and place. Tell them to remind each other. Offer to give them a call the night before the meeting.

4 Provide a way for youth to contact you if they need to and remind them that they can use the Question Box.

5 *Optional:* If you are using the all-day retreat option for Session 6, pass out permission slips. Ask youth to return them at the start of the next session.

Skills Building: Communication

Purpose	Youth will learn communication and negotiation skills to assist in carrying out responsible decisions.

Session Overview
(95 minutes)

1 **Opening Ritual and Review** (15 minutes)

2 **SODA Decision-Making Model: Step 4** (10 minutes)

3 **Communication Game: Changing Messages** (10 minutes)

4 **Communication Styles: Aggressive, Assertive and Nonassertive** (25 minutes)

5 **Communicating Without Words** (10 minutes)

6 **Sex: A Decision for Two** (20 minutes)

7 **Wrap-Up and Closing Ritual** (5 minutes)

Preparation

Pre-Session Activities

❏ Read over and become familiar with Session 5 activities.

❏ Prepare snacks.

❏ Copy **Communication Styles** worksheet for each participant. (See page 124.)

Materials

❏ snacks

❏ Family Tree, Groundrules, SODA Model and Field Assignment charts

❏ masking tape

❏ Field Assignment worksheets from Session 3

❏ newsprint and markers

❏ props for Communication Styles activity

❏ **Communication Styles** worksheet, 1 for each participant

I. Opening Ritual and Review

☺ **Objective:**	Youth will review highlights from Session 4.
🕐 **Time:**	15 minutes
✂ **Materials:**	None

Procedure

1 After the opening ritual, sit down with youth and remind them of groundrules.

2 Answer any questions from the Question Box.

3 Review Session 4 by asking the following questions:

- What are the steps for putting on a condom?

- Where can you get information about STD?

- What are some guidelines for approaching an adult to talk about sex?

4 Ask if any youth completed field assignments. Have volunteers share what they did and what they learned from their assignments.

5 *Optional:* Collect permission slips for the all-day retreat, if you are using the option for Session 6.

2.

SODA Decision-Making Model—Step 4: Action

Source: S. Schinke, A. Gordon and R. Weston. 1990. Self-Instruction to Prevent HIV Infection Among African-American and Hispanic-American Adolescents. Journal of Consulting and Clinical Psychology 58 (4): 432-436.

☺ **Objective:**   Youth will acquire skills for decision making, with a focus on Step 4: Action.

🕐 **Time:**   10 minutes

✂ **Materials:**   Newsprint and markers

SODA Model and Family Tree charts

Procedure

1 Briefly review the first 3 steps of decision making.

Step 1: Stop—**Stop and state the problem.** Pause and give yourself time to decide what the problem really is.

Step 2: Options—**Consider the options** or choices and the consequences of those choices. Educate yourself so you know all the choices and consequences before you make a decision.

Step 3: Decide—**Decide and choose the best solution** from the options. What is best will vary depending on the problem and your values (strongly held beliefs). Making a decision is done by weighing the advantages and disadvantages of the options.

Explain that today, they are going to work on Step 4—Action.

Step 4: Action—**Act on your decision.** Once a decision is made, it must be put into action. To accomplish this, you may need to learn new skills for communication, negotiation or other skills related to carrying out the decision (e.g., condom use, use of birth control).

2 Lead a discussion using 1 or 2 of the following options from the last session. Explain that in an earlier session they looked at what options

Chantel/Tavon might choose because of her/his values. Now they will look at what skills she/he might need to act on the decision. Examples:

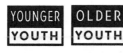

- Option 1: If Chantel/Tavon decided not to have sex, what kind of skills would she/he need?

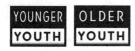

- Option 2: If Chantel/Tavon decided to have sex, what kind of skills would she/he need?

- Option 3: If she/he decided to tell their boyfriend/girlfriend that they had to use condoms what skills would she/he need?

Write the skills on newsprint as youth identify them. Be sure to add the following skills to the list if youth do not mention them:

- communication skills

- listening skills

- negotiating skills (how to communicate what you want)

- must know how to use whatever method of protection she/he decides to use

- must know how to use a condom

State that today they will practice some of these skills.

Notes for Group Leaders: Keep this discussion as fast paced as possible. You only need to focus on 1 or 2 options and have youth identify the skills. Try to make it as interactive as possible.

3.

Communication Game: Changing Messages

☺ **Objective:**   Youth will learn the consequences of gossiping and the importance of not making assumptions.

🕐 **Time:**   10 minutes

✂ **Materials:**   None

Procedure

1 Have youth sit in a circle. Group leaders should join them in the circle.

2 One of the group leaders should whisper to the youth on his or her right a very brief, positive story with names and places that have some interest to the group.

3 Ask this first youth to pass the story on by whispering it to the person sitting next to him or her. Continue to pass the story around the entire circle in this way.

4 After everyone has been told the story, have the last youth recite the story that she or he heard, and then compare it to the original one.

5 If time permits, give each youth the opportunity of starting a new story. Remind them it must be a *positive* story. For example, My favorite (pet, friend, teacher) is _____ because...(not, for example, saying "so and so is ugly," etc.).

6 Lead a discussion using the following questions:

- What happened to the message? Why?

- Does this ever happen in everyday life?

- What can be some of the problems when people gossip?

- What can you do to minimize the problems that occur from gossiping?

7 Remind youth that miscommunication is a common problem. This is especially true when they gossip. They should always be careful of the source of their information. Let them know that they will continue to work on skills to improve their communication in this session and the next.

4. Communication Styles: Aggressive, Assertive and Nonassertive

☺ **Objective:** Youth will learn and practice effective communication skills.

🕐 **Time:** 25 minutes

✄ **Materials:** Roleplay props: pizza restaurant hat or apron, tie for shoe store sales person, shoes, etc.

Communication Styles worksheet, 1 for each participant

Procedure

1 Choose a volunteer to be "Al Bundy," the shoe salesperson. The group leader will play a customer who is returning a pair of shoes because they had a hole in them.

2 Perform the first roleplay. Play an exaggerated "passive" person. Look down at the ground, try to get Al's attention in a barely audible voice, barely state the problem and don't offer any solution. More than likely "Al" will not give you a new pair of shoes, then leave the store quietly.

3 Ask:

- How was I acting?
- What was my voice like?
- Did I tell Al what I wanted (a new pair of shoes)?
- Did I get what I wanted?
- Where were my eyes?
- What was my body like?

4 Repeat the roleplay. This time play an "assertive" person. In a clear voice, looking right at "Al," explain that you were in the day before and bought a pair of shoes, but they have a hole in them and you would like to exchange them for a new pair. You have your receipt.

More than likely, "Al" will give you a new pair of shoes. If he doesn't, politely ask for the manager. Have another youth play the manager and repeat the above scenario. Leave with your new pair of shoes.

5 Again ask youth the questions in Step 3.

6 The third time, play an "aggressive" person. Go into the store yelling and screaming out of control. Don't give "Al" a chance to respond. Storm out of the store exclaiming you will never shop there again.

7 Ask youth the questions in Step 3.

8 Ask which method gave you the results you wanted—to have the shoes exchanged. Tell youth that **assertive** behavior is more likely to get us what we want in a way that is respectful of others.

9 Distribute and review the **Communication Styles** worksheet.

10 Have youth break up into groups of 2 or 3 and roleplay the different roles themselves. Have one be the customer, one be an employee and one be the manager of a pizza store. The customer asked for a pizza with no meat on it and received a pizza with meat. If time allows, you can have one or more groups do the roleplay in front of the group.

11 Discuss the roleplay using the following questions:

- What behavior worked to get the results the customer wanted?
- Are there times when someone should be aggressive? (e.g., sports, when life is in danger)
- Are there times when someone should be passive?

Notes for Group Leaders: This exercise may bring up issues of cultural differences in communication styles. Explain that in some cultures an action might be perceived as aggressive while in another culture it might be perceived as assertive. People have to look at the circumstances to determine the best way to communicate. It's important to be sensitive to the other person's reaction. If the other person reacts negatively, you may need to find another way to communicate.

Have examples of the 3 types of behavior to share so youth don't get confused.

Worksheet

Communication Styles

	Nonassertive (Timid or shy)	Assertive (Strong)	Aggressive (Bossy)
Content	often unclear nonspecific indirect	clear specific direct problem-oriented suggested solution	nonspecific, especially in terms of outcome directed against the other
Voice	soft trailing off	clear moderate in tone	usually loud, harsh
Facial expression	avoidance of eye contact, eyes downcast	eye contact	glaring
Posture	bent over fidgety	erect comfortable	rigid tense
Your feelings	shy anxious scared	confident self-respecting comfortable	self-righteous angry
The other's feelings	confused unclear	respected	hurt angry
Goal of the Behavior	avoid conflict	a change in the situation; a change in the other's behavior	put the other person down

5.

Communicating Without Words

Source: Adapted from P. Kramer. 1990. The Dynamics of Relationships.

☺ **Objective:** Youth will understand how important our nonverbal messages can be and how difficult they can be to interpret.

🕐 **Time:** 10 minutes

✂ **Materials:** None

Procedure

1 Have the group stand in a line, all facing the same direction. Explain and demonstrate how the game works.

Tell them you are going to secretly give the person at the end of the line a particular action or emotion to nonverbally pass on to the person in front of her or him. This person will tap the person in front of her or him on the shoulder. When the second person turns around so that they are facing each other, person 1 will attempt to pass on the action or emotion nonverbally.

When person 2 thinks she or he knows what the emotion is, person 2 will turn back around and tap the next person in line on the shoulder. Person 2 will now attempt to nonverbally pass on the action or emotion to person 3. The process continues until the last person in line has been tapped and received the action or emotion from the previous person.

Play the game.

Possible actions or emotions to use:

- flirting with someone
- refusing something
- trying to tell someone you like him/her
- feeling sad
- feeling angry
- feeling happy

2 Ask the last person in line to report to the group what she or he thinks the action or emotion was. Most likely she or he will not know because of a miscommunication somewhere along the way.

This exercise can show youth how often our gestures and facial expressions say something that we may not be saying with words. Reinforce that they need to pay just as much attention to their nonverbal as their verbal messages. Explain that we also need to pay attention to what others are saying with their body language. Even when we are not talking we may still be saying something.

3 Lead a discussion about the activity using the following questions:

- Was it difficult to figure out what the other person was doing?

- What can happen if someone doesn't understand what the other person is trying to say under these circumstances?

- How can you be sure you have understood the person you are communicating with? (*Note:* This is a key point! The group leaders should give some examples of how to "check out" communications before reacting, e.g., "Are you saying that...?" "I'm not sure I understand, what do you mean?" Emphasize that we need both verbal and nonverbal communication to send and receive clear messages.)

- Do you think boys and girls ever give each other confusing messages? Can you think of an example?

- How can you tell if someone is making a pass at you?

- How can a person tell someone "yes" or "no" without saying anything?

Emphasize again how important clear communication is—youth need to make sure they are sending clear verbal and nonverbal messages and understanding others. The next activity shows some of the problems that can occur when communication breaks down.

Notes for Group Leaders: This lesson could also be taught by playing charades if that is easier.

6.

Sex: A Decision for Two

Source: P. Brick, C. Charlton, H. Kunins and S. Brown. 1989. Teaching Safer Sex. Hackensack, NJ: The Center for Family Life Education, Planned Parenthood of Bergen County, Inc.

☺ **Objective:** Youth will understand how date rape occurs and identify ways to prevent it.

🕐 **Time:** 20 minutes

✂ **Materials:** **Yvonne's Story** (See page 130.)

Procedure

1 Introduce the activity by stating that often poor communication just results in misunderstandings or hurt feelings but sometimes it can have more serious consequences like what happens in the story I want to tell you.

2 Read youth **Yvonne's Story.**

3 Lead a discussion about the story using the following questions:

• Identify 3 times during the story when John did not respect Yvonne's feelings.

• Identify 3 times during the story when Yvonne left herself unprotected.

• If John were sensitive to his partner, what signals would have told him that Yvonne did not want to continue?

• If Yvonne had been more forceful, what 3 things could she have said to make her real feelings clear to John?

Explain that date rape often proceeds through 3 stages:

• **Stage 1.** Someone (usually the male) enters the other's "personal space" in a public place (kissing, hand on breast or thigh, etc.). Ask: When did this happen in the story?

- **Stage 2.** The partner does not forcefully stop this intrusion and the aggressor assumes it's OK. Ask: When did this happen in the story?

- **Stage 3.** The aggressor gets the couple to a secluded place where the rape takes place. Ask: When did this happen in the story?

4 Ask youth what kind of communication style Yvonne was using. What about John? Remind youth of the importance of using an assertive communication style to make sure others understand what you are trying to tell them.

5 Tell youth that some people have misunderstandings about what rape is or how it happens. Tell them you'd like to clarify any misunderstandings they may have by asking if certain statements are myth or fact.

Read each of the following statements and ask youth to state if it is myth or fact. Correct any misinformation.

- Rape is committed by strangers. (*Myth. Over half of all reported rapes are committed by a person known by the victim.*)

- If a boyfriend/girlfriend forces someone to have sex, it is rape. (*Fact.*)

- Rape only occurs outdoors in dark alleys. (*Myth. Over half of all rapes occur in either the victim's or assailant's home.*)

- Rape is caused by the way the girl dresses or acts. (*Myth.* **This is an excuse.** *Everyone has the right to decide with whom he or she will or will not have sex. No one has the right to have sex with anyone against his or her will no matter what the situation.*)

- It is better not to tell anyone if you are raped. (*Myth. Whether a person decides to report to the police or not, the services of a sexual assault center are available in most communities 24 hours a day. People who keep their thoughts and feelings bottled up inside are more likely to have long-lasting negative effects from the rape.*)

- Child sexual abuse is rare, happens out of the blue and is usually an extreme form of child abuse. *(Myth. This form of abuse develops gradually over a period of time and usually will be repeated unless it is stopped. Although the forms of abuse may become more serious as time goes on, the majority are not the torture/murder types seen on TV.)*

6 Make sure the youth have a number they can use if they are ever assaulted or want to talk to someone about sexual assault.

- National Sexual Assault Hotline: 1-800-656-HOPE(4673)

- National Youth Crisis Hotline: 1-800-422-4453

Notes for Group Leaders: This activity might lead to youth disclosing that they have been victims of date rape or sexual abuse. Be sure you know both your agency policies on such disclosures and local counseling and support resources to recommend for youth.

Yvonne's Story

8:00 p.m. "Hurry up," urged Yvonne, "I thought you said Willie would meet us downstairs at 8:00 p.m."

Jill, Yvonne's best friend, replied, "Yeah, I know. Listen, I forgot to mention it—but that guy you know from Booker T is gonna come with us. You remember? He's a good friend of Willie's."

Yvonne suddenly felt nervous. "You mean John? You know I think he's really fine. What do I say?"

Jill answered, "Just act natural." Yvonne nodded, thinking that the party was going to be really good with John there.

8:15 At the party, John paid a lot of attention to Yvonne. She was thrilled. They started to dance. Yvonne knew she was a terrific dancer and she loved to dance, especially with a fine guy like John. They spent about two hours together, alternating between talking and dancing.

10:30 A slow song came on and John immediately pulled Yvonne close. Yvonne didn't feel entirely comfortable dancing in this way, but she didn't say anything. Instead, she put her hands on his chest to keep their bodies from pressing too close.

John was really enjoying himself. He'd noticed Yvonne in the neighborhood and thought she was attractive. He couldn't believe his luck. He felt he was acting so smooth and charming. He could sense she was responding to it. He decided to kiss her.

Yvonne was surprised by John's kiss. She was attracted to him, but felt uncomfortable that he was kissing her in public. She didn't want him to think that she didn't like him so she just tilted her head down to end the kiss. John thought to himself: She really likes me. She's snuggling in after that kiss.

11:00 The dance floor became packed again as the music got fast. Yvonne felt slightly dizzy from the dancing and wanted to sit down. John was worried by Yvonne's mood change. He felt very turned on and wanted to be alone with her. He said, "Want to go outside for some air? It's pretty stuffy in here."

Yvonne's Story (continued)

Yvonne looked around for Jill but didn't see her. She said to John, "OK, but just for a little while." She felt nervous about being alone with him, but she also felt silly about feeling that way.

11:10 Once outside, John put his arm around Yvonne and began kissing her. He was thinking how much she wanted to be kissed since she had been dancing so sexy all evening. Yvonne, still unsure of what she wanted, pulled away and began talking about how much she liked middle school. John thought she was talkative because she was excited. So he continued to kiss her. Yvonne again pulled away and stood up saying, "I think I should get going. Let's find Jill."

11:30 John followed Yvonne back inside to the party. They found out that Jill had just left with Willie. John offered to walk Yvonne home, thinking he could spend some more time with her alone. Yvonne agreed.

12:00 When they arrived at Yvonne's house, John asked, "Isn't your Mom here?" Yvonne told him her mom was on a date. John thought to himself: Yvonne wants to be alone with me too. That's why she brought me back here. John said to Yvonne, "Let's go inside then. We don't have to say goodnight out here." Yvonne hesitated. She told John that she was very tired and wanted to go to sleep. John said, "I won't stay long." He took her key from her hand and opened the door. When Yvonne stood in the hall and said goodnight, John laughed. He walked past her into the living room saying, "Come sit for awhile." He motioned to the space next to him on the couch.

12:10 Yvonne sat down, tired and confused, and began to explain once again that she was tired and John should stay only for a few minutes. John, thinking how sexy Yvonne was, moved over and began to kiss her. He pushed her down onto the couch and began to unbutton her shirt. Yvonne did not respond to his kisses and pushed him away muttering, "No, stop." John ignored her. He continued to undress both of them, thinking she really wanted it.

Yvonne stopped saying no and began to cry when John began to rape her.

7. Wrap-Up and Closing Ritual

☺ **Objective:**	Youth will provide feedback on Session 5 and summarize what they have learned.
🕐 **Time:**	5 minutes
✄ **Materials:**	None

Procedure

1 Have group sit in a circle. Perform the chosen closing ritual.

2 Gather feedback about the day's session by asking the following questions:

- What did they like?
- What didn't they like?
- What did they learn?
- What would they like to learn more about at another session?

3 Remind youth of the next meeting time and place. Tell them to remind each other. Offer to give them a call the night before the meeting.

4 Provide a way for youth to contact you if they need to and remind them that they can use the Question Box.

5 *Optional:* If you are using the all-day retreat option for Session 6, remind youth of the day for the retreat and the time and place to meet. Review any logistics, such as where the bus will pick them up.

Remind youth that:

- They should wear something comfortable and weather appropriate.
- They do not need to bring money.
- They *must* bring their permission slip, if they have not already returned it.

Information About Sexual Health

Purpose	Youth will learn information about sexual health.

Session Overview
(100 minutes)

1 Opening Ritual and Review (15 minutes)

2 Ways to Show You Care (20 minutes)

3 HIV Transmission Game (15 minutes)

4 Contraception Lesson (45 minutes)

5 Wrap-Up and Closing Ritual (5 minutes)

Notes for Group Leaders: See the Resource Section, page 183, for the all-day retreat option for Session 6. If you choose this option, be sure to prepare for the retreat as described on pages 187–188 in addition to your preparation for Session 6.

Preparation

**Pre-Session
Activities**

❏ Read over and become familiar with Session 6 activities.

❏ Prepare snacks.

❏ Make "With or Without Intercourse" and "Intercourse Only" signs.
(See samples on pages 138 and 139.)

Materials

❏ marked index cards and pencils for HIV transmission game
(See Activity 3 for specific instructions.)

❏ pencils, 1 for each participant

❏ newsprint

❏ blank cardboard and newsprint

❏ markers

❏ snacks

❏ Field Assignment chart and worksheets from Session 3

❏ 8-1/2" x 11" sheets of paper or 3" x 5" cards with Reasons to Have
Sex written on them (See Activity 2.)

❏ "With or Without Intercourse" and "Intercourse Only" signs

❏ samples of birth control methods (condom, female condom, foam,
diaphragm, spermicidal jelly and birth control pills) and male/female
anatomy models for contraception lesson (See Activity 4.)

I.

Opening Ritual and Review

☺ **Objective:**	Youth will review highlights from Session 5.
🕐 **Time:**	15 minutes
✂ **Materials:**	None

Procedure

1 After the opening ritual, have youth share any new field assignments they have done.

2 Answer any questions from the Question Box.

3 Review Session 5 by asking the following questions:

- What is the difference between assertive and aggressive behavior?

- Why is assertive behavior often a good choice?

- What is nonverbal communication?

- What are ways to protect yourself from date rape? (Girls)

- If a girl says NO she means NO. Why should the boy believe her? (Boys)

2.

Ways to Show You Care

Source: P. Brick, C. Charlton, H. Kunins and S. Brown. 1989. Teaching Safer Sex. Hackensack, NJ: The Center for Family Life Education, Planned Parenthood of Bergen County, Inc.

☺ **Objective:** Youth will discover that positive feelings usually associated with sexual intercourse can also be experienced without intercourse and will recognize the importance of "Showing Ways You Care" as a safer sex option.

🕐 **Time:** 20 minutes

✂ **Materials:** 8-1/2" x 11" pieces of paper

newsprint and markers

Signs that say "With or Without Intercourse" and "Intercourse Only"

☑ **Preparation:** Write each of the following Reasons to Have Sex on an 8-1/2" x 11" piece of paper:

- have special body feelings
- have an orgasm
- feel close to a partner
- show partner your love
- get pregnant
- feel like a man/woman

- be sexually satisfied
- feel sexy
- feel horny
- feel loved
- have fun
- be normal

Procedure

1 Write on newsprint: THE LARGEST ORGAN OF PLEASURE IS…. Ask youth to complete the sentence. Accept all answers. Finally, if it has not been suggested, tell them it's the skin—we really are "sexy" all over.

2 Write: THE MOST IMPORTANT SEX ORGAN IS…. Again, ask for responses. Note that most sexologists believe it's the brain, because the brain has learned what is considered "sexy" in this particular society.

3 Ask for definitions of intercourse that may include vaginal, oral and anal intercourse. Note that in our society when people say "having sex" they are usually referring to genital sex, i.e., intercourse.

4 Ask youth to brainstorm the reasons people have intercourse. Write each reason on an 8-1/2" x 11" piece of paper. Add these to the "Reasons" you prepared earlier.

5 Tape the signs "With or Without Intercourse" and "Intercourse Only" on different sides of the room. Ask for volunteers to select a reason and tape it under the correct sign.

6 If youth put any cards under the "Intercourse Only" sign ask why. Do others agree? Ask: Is it important that people can experience many of the pleasures of intercourse without actually having intercourse?

(*Note*: Almost all feelings/consequences are possible with or without intercourse, even pregnancy through artificial insemination.)

7 State that there are other ways to be close to a person and show you care without having sexual intercourse. Ask youth to brainstorm ways to be close. The list may include holding hands, hugging, body massage, bathing together, masturbation, sensuous feeding, fantasizing, watching erotic movies, reading erotic books and magazines, making or giving a gift, going to a movie together, writing notes, etc.

8 Write ADVANTAGES AND DISADVANTAGES on newsprint. Ask youth to brainstorm the advantages and disadvantages of showing you care without having sexual intercourse as compared with having intercourse. Be sure to include good ways to protect against unwanted pregnancy and HIV/STD.

9 Summarize by saying that it's normal to want to experience intimacy, closeness and sexual pleasure. However, it is important to do it in a way that is safe and healthy. Point out that, as they have seen, there are many ways to do this without having sex.

With
or
Without
Intercourse

Sample Sign

Intercourse Only

3.

HIV Transmission Game

Source: Adapted from Center for Population Options' Guide to Implementing TAP (Teens for AIDS Prevention Peer Education Program).

☺ **Objective:** Youth will have increased awareness of how quickly HIV and other STD can be spread and how they can be prevented.

🕐 **Time:** 15 minutes

✂ **Materials:** Prepared index cards and pencils, 1 for each participant

☑ **Preparation:** Prepare the index cards by marking 1 card with a small "x" on the upper right corner and about 10% of the cards with a small "c." Mark 1 or 2 cards with "Do not participate. Do not talk to anyone. Do not sign anyone's card and do not let anyone sign your card."

Procedure

Note: You need at least 15 people to play this game. Recruit other youth or adults if you do not have enough people in the group.

1 Distribute 1 index card to each youth. Tell them that a few of the cards have special instructions and that people should keep the special instructions on their cards secret for the next few minutes. Ask youth to stand and introduce themselves to 3 people and ask each of those people to sign their card. Each person should get 3 signatures from other people. Once they have 3 names on the card they should sit down.

2 When everyone has collected 3 signatures and is sitting, ask the person with the "x" on his or her card to stand up. Say that you are sorry, but the lab results have come back and he or she has HIV.

Ask everyone with that person's name on his or her card to stand up. Tell them you regret to tell them that they have been exposed to HIV, and should go to the clinic to be tested. Ask everyone who has the name of a standing person on his or her card to stand up. Let them know that they too have been exposed to HIV. Continue this process until everyone is standing except for the designated nonparticipators.

3 Ask youth to check if they had a "c" marked on their card. These people used a condom and were not at significant risk. Have these youth sit down.

4 Remind youth that this activity is "pretend" and only a demonstration. Stress that HIV is not spread by casual contact and that these youth do not really have HIV. Explain that HIV is only spread by exchanging body fluids (blood, semen, vaginal fluids, breastmilk) through sexual contact, by sharing needles, or from a mother to her unborn child.

5 Lead a discussion using the following questions:

- How did the person with the "x" feel? How did you feel toward person "x"?

- What were the initial feelings of those of you who weren't allowed to play? How did those feelings change during the course of the activity? How did the group feel about the nonparticipants at first? How about later?

- What makes it difficult not to participate in an activity that everyone else is doing?

- How did the people who discovered they had used condoms feel?

- Person "x" did not know he or she was infected. How could we have known ahead of time?

6 Summarize the following points from the activity:

- You can't tell if someone is infected with HIV.

- If you have sexual intercourse or share needles with someone with HIV you can become infected.

- If you choose to have sexual intercourse, it is important to use a latex condom to protect yourself from HIV and other STD.

- If you choose to have sexual intercourse you should limit your number of partners.

- Although it is difficult not to do what everyone else is doing, sometimes it is the best thing.

Notes for Group Leaders: Youth can get loud during this activity and you may need to keep the noise from escalating. A relatively large number of youth (about 15-20) are needed to make this game work.

---

4. Contraception Lesson

<table>
<tr><td>☺ Objective:</td><td>Youth will learn about the various methods of contraception.</td></tr>
<tr><td>🕐 Time:</td><td>45 minutes</td></tr>
<tr><td>✂ Materials:</td><td>Samples of birth control pills, foam, diaphragm, spermicidal jelly, condom, female condom, male model (or a cucumber), female pelvic anatomy model</td></tr>
<tr><td>☑ Preparation:</td><td>Be familiar with all the information on the various methods of birth control to ensure that you will be able to answer youths' questions.</td></tr>
</table>

Procedure

1 Begin by displaying all the birth control methods. Overview each of the methods using the information sheets provided.

2 **Overview of Barrier Methods:** Hold up the condom, female condom, foam and diaphragm. Explain that these are called "barrier methods." What that means is that they block, or act like a barrier to stop the sperm from reaching the egg.

With the pelvic model, show how the egg comes down from the ovary through the fallopian tube and into the uterus. Explain that in the fallopian tube it is possible for the sperm and egg to meet and for the woman to become pregnant. Barrier methods act to stop this from happening. State that only "condoms" offer any protection from HIV or STD.

Explain each barrier method in greater detail using the information sheets provided on pages 145–148.

3 **Overview of Hormonal Methods:** Hold up the sample of birth control pills. Explain that there are also "hormonal methods" of birth control.

These include birth control pills, Norplant™ and Depo Provera (the shot). These methods stop a woman's body from releasing an egg each month and change the lining of her uterus so an egg cannot grow there. These methods do not stop sperm from entering the woman's body, and they do *not* protect from HIV or other STD. Explain the various hormonal methods in greater detail using the information sheets provided on pages 149–152.

4 Summarize for youth by stating that when thinking about which birth control method to use they should consider the following:

- Their lifestyle

- Their values

- Side effects

- How regularly do they have sex?

- Are they comfortable touching themselves?

- The effectiveness of the method

- Protection from HIV and other STD

Notes for Group Leaders: Most youth are very interested in this session. For more information on contraception see *Contraceptive Technology* (R.A. Hatcher et al. 1998. 17th ed. New York: Ardent Media) or *The New Our Bodies, Ourselves* (The Boston Women's Health Book Collective. 1992. New York: Simon and Schuster).

Information Sheet

Condom

The condom goes over a man's penis and stops the sperm from getting inside the woman. The latex condom is the most important method of birth control because it also stops the transmission of HIV and other sexually transmitted disease (STD).

Condoms can be bought without a doctor's prescription at any drugstore. Many clinics give them away for free.

You should only use a water-based lubricant (e.g., KY Jelly™) with a condom. Oil-based lubricants (oil, Vaseline™, lotion) will destroy a condom.

Advantages

- No prescription is necessary.

- You can find condoms for free or at low cost at many clinics.

- Protects against pregnancy *and* HIV and other STD.

Disadvantages/Side Effects

- There are generally no side effects or risks from using condoms.

- Occasionally, people are allergic to chemicals in the spermicide. You can switch brands if you or your partner is allergic.

- Condoms may decrease spontaneity and sometimes some people are uncomfortable using them. Talking about them before sex and practicing can help!

Information Sheet

Female Condom

The female condom goes inside the woman's vagina and keeps the sperm and egg from meeting. The female condom is a polyurethane pouch that has a ring at each end. One ring goes inside the woman's body and covers her cervix. The other ring, at the open end of the tube, hangs outside the woman's body. Like the male condom, the female condom stops the transmission of HIV and other sexually transmitted disease (STD).

Female condoms can be bought without a doctor's prescription at any drugstore. Some clinics give them away for free, although these are harder to find because the female condoms cost close to a dollar each.

Only water-based lubricants should be used with the female condom. Oil-based lubricants (oil, Vaseline™, lotion) will destroy a condom.

The male and female condom should *not* be used together because one or both will not stay in place.

Advantages

- No prescription is necessary.

- Protects against pregnancy *and* HIV and other STD.

- The woman has more control over condom use.

Disadvantages/Side Effects

- There are generally no side effects or risks from using condoms.

- Occasionally, people are allergic to chemicals in the spermicide.

- A woman must be comfortable touching her body to insert the condom.

- Part of the condom hangs outside the woman's body. This might be uncomfortable for some women.

- Condoms may decrease spontaneity and sometimes some people are uncomfortable using them. Talking about them before sex and practicing can help!

Information Sheet

Foam

Since condoms are not 100% effective, there are some things you can do to make it even less likely a pregnancy will occur. One of these things is to use spermicidal foam with the condom.

To use foam *(show the container)*, shake it about 20 times. Then use the applicator to put the foam (about 2 applicators full) inside the woman's vagina. *(Show using the model, but don't actually put the foam in the model!)* The foam should be put in 20 minutes before sex. You need to put in more foam if you have intercourse again.

The foam acts as an extra security. In case the condom breaks, foam will kill the sperm. Do not douche for at least 6 hours after intercourse. It takes that long for the foam to kill all of the sperm.

Foam should always be used with a condom. Foam is not very effective on its own.

Advantages

- No prescription is necessary. Contraceptive foam can be purchased at any drugstore.

- Provides extra protection from pregnancy when used with condoms.

Disadvantages/Side Effects

- There are generally no side effects or risks from using foam.

- Occasionally, people are allergic to chemicals in the foam. If either partner becomes allergic, try switching to a different brand.

- It does not protect you against HIV and STD.

Diaphragm

You must go see a doctor or nurse to get fitted and prescribed a diaphragm. It comes in different sizes.

You have to use a spermicidal jelly or cream with the diaphragm. Put approximately 1 tablespoon of jelly in the diaphragm and spread it around with a finger. The woman then inserts the diaphragm in her vagina and places it over her cervix. She should check to make sure the diaphragm is placed over the cervix (the cervix feels like the tip of your nose).

The diaphragm blocks the sperm from getting to the egg. The diaphragm does not protect from sexually transmitted disease because the vagina is not covered, so there can be an exchange of blood and sexual fluids. A condom must be used with the diaphragm to protect you from HIV and other STD.

If a woman has sex more than one time, she must put more spermicide in. This is done using an applicator. *(Demonstrate this with the model.)* A woman also needs to put in more spermicide if it has been more than 2 hours since she inserted the diaphragm.

The diaphragm must stay in for at least 6 hours after the woman has sex to make sure that all the sperm are killed. After 6 hours she needs to reach inside and use her finger to bring the diaphragm out. She then rinses it off with soap and water and stores it. The diaphragm can be used again and again.

Advantages

- You can put it in up to 2 hours before you have sex and not worry about it.
- You are not putting any hormones into your body.

Disadvantages/Side Effects

- You must be comfortable touching your body.
- It does not protect you completely against HIV and other STD. You must also use a latex condom.

Other Considerations

- Practice inserting, wearing and removing the diaphragm before you use it.

Information Sheet

Birth Control Pills

Probably one of the most common methods of birth control is the birth control pill. There are lots of different kinds of birth control pills. For a woman to begin taking pills she must go to the doctor and get a prescription. The doctor will look at her age, weight, medical history, etc., and prescribe the best pill for her.

The birth control pill works in 2 ways: (1) The pill causes a woman to stop releasing an egg, so she can't get pregnant, and (2) it also changes the lining of her uterus so that if an egg does get released it will not be able to implant itself in the uterus.

The birth control pill is probably one of the most effective methods for a woman to not get pregnant. But it does not protect her at all from sexually transmitted disease, including HIV. So even if the woman is on the pill, she should still have her partner use a condom.

A woman begins taking the pill on the first Sunday after her period. It's best to take the pill at approximately the same time every day. This is easiest on the body and also gives the best protection against pregnancy. A woman needs to have taken an entire pack of pills before she is protected against pregnancy, so it is very important to use another method of birth control for the first month. Even after that first month it is important to continue to use condoms to protect against HIV and other sexually transmitted disease.

When a woman first goes on the pill she sometimes experiences some minor side effects. Some common side effects are breast swelling or tenderness, spotting between periods, depression, weight gain, nausea and skin changes, such as breaking out. Most of these side effects go away after a woman's body adjusts to being on the pill. If the side effects are really bad or don't go away after 3 months, she should go back to the doctor and discuss switching to a different kind of pill.

There are 2 different ways pills are taken. One is called the 28-day pack. With these pills you take 1 pill every day until all the pills are gone. At the end of the pack there are 7 pills that are a different color. It is while taking these pills that you get your period. As soon as you finish the pack you begin to take pills from the next pack. There are also pills that are in a 21-day pack. With these pills, after you finish the last

(continued)

Information Sheet

(Birth Control Pills, continued)

pill you wait 1 week before starting a new pack. During this week you get your period.

Some women miss a period when they are on the pill. If you have been taking your pills correctly, you shouldn't worry too much. But if you've missed more than 1 pill it is probably a good idea to get a pregnancy test. If a woman misses 2 periods, she should get a pregnancy test. If she is not pregnant she might want to discuss with her doctor changing the kind of pill she is on.

It is important that women know that if they miss any more than 1 pill they could get pregnant. You should use another method of birth control, such as a condom, if you miss 2 pills in a month.

Advantages

- When taken properly, the pill is one of the most effective temporary methods of birth control.
- The pill does not interrupt sex.
- Periods are generally shorter and lighter with less cramping.

Disadvantages

- Birth control pills give no protection against HIV and other STD.
- Some common side effects include breast swelling or tenderness, spotting between periods, depression, weight gain, nausea, and skin changes such as breaking out.
- Some women are not able to take the pill because of medical reasons.

Other Considerations

- You should always let medical providers know that you are on the pill.
- Some other drugs may make the pill less effective. Your medical provider can let you know.
- If you become ill and have several days of vomiting and/or diarrhea, use another method of birth control in addition to the pill.

Information Sheet

Norplant™

Norplant is a type of birth control that works similar to birth control pills. Norplant™ looks like 6 little match sticks that are implanted in a woman's arm. Instead of taking a pill every day, the implants release small amounts of the hormone into the woman's body. With Norplant™ a woman is protected against pregnancy for 5 years.

Norplant™ is one of the most effective methods of birth control. Unfortunately, like birth control pills, Norplant™ gives no protection against HIV and other STD, so a condom should be used with Norplant™ at all times.

The Norplant™ system placement usually takes about 15 minutes. A woman is given a local anesthetic, so she feels little or no pain.

The most common side effect reported is that women's periods become irregular. They may last longer, and there might be occasional bleeding or spotting between periods. Sometimes a woman will not get a period for several months. Other possible side effects include headache, nausea, nervousness and dizziness.

There are some other possible risks with both birth control pills and Norplant™ that should be discussed with a doctor.

Advantages

- Norplant™ is one of the most effective methods of birth control.
- It does not interrupt sex.
- You do not have to remember to take a pill every day.

Disadvantages/Side Effects

- Many woman have irregular periods while on Norplant™
- Some women experience headaches, nausea, nervousness and dizziness.
- Norplant™ lasts for 5 years and it is sometimes difficult to find someone to remove it.
- Norplant™ gives no protection against HIV and other STD.

Information Sheet

Depo-Provera (The Shot)

Depo-Provera is a shot a woman gets from a doctor or nurse every 3 months. When taken as scheduled—4 times a year or every 3 months—it is more than 99% effective.

A woman must receive the first injection during the first 5 days of a normal menstrual period. When administered in this way, she is protected from pregnancy immediately after she receives the injection.

Advantages

- The shot is one of the most effective methods of birth control.
- It does not interrupt sex.
- You do not have to remember to take a pill every day.

Disadvantages/Side Effects

- Most women experience weight gain and irregular or unpredictable menstrual bleeding.
- After 1 year of use, many women stop having periods altogether.
- Some women who use it experience nervousness, dizziness, stomach discomfort, headaches or fatigue.
- The shot gives no protection against HIV and other STD.

5.

Wrap-Up and Closing Ritual

☺ **Objective:** Youth will provide feedback on Session 6 and summarize what they have learned.

🕐 **Time:** 5 minutes

✂ **Materials:** None

Procedure

1 Have the group sit in a circle. Perform the chosen closing ritual.

2 Gather feedback about the day's session by asking the following questions:

- What did they like?

- What didn't they like?

- What did they learn?

- What would they like to learn more about at another session?

3 Remind youth of the next meeting time and place. Tell them to remind each other. Offer to give them a call the night before the meeting.

4 Provide a way for youth to contact you if they need to and remind them that they can use the Question Box.

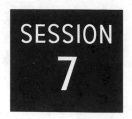

Attitudes and Skills for Sexual Health

Purpose	Youth will learn attitudes and skills that support sexual health.

Session Overview
(85 minutes)

1 **Opening Ritual and Review** (10 minutes)

2 **Goal Setting: My Future** (20 minutes)

3 **Images of Sex** (30 minutes)

4 **Roleplay: Saying NO or Asking to Use a Condom** (20 minutes)

5 **Wrap-Up and Closing Ritual** (5 minutes)

Preparation

Pre-Session Activities

❏ Read over and become familiar with Session 7 activities.

❏ Prepare snacks.

❏ Prepare **Adjustments to the Future** cards. (See page 160.)

Materials

❏ snacks

❏ pieces of colored 8-1/2" x 11" paper, 3 for each participant

❏ small pieces of paper or index cards for Images of Sex activity

❏ a box of crayons, newsprint, markers, pens, tape and scissors for each small group

❏ Groundrules and Field Assignment charts

❏ Field Assignment worksheets from Session 3

❏ props for the roleplay

❏ **Adjustments to the Future** cards

1. Opening Ritual and Review

☺ **Objective:**	Youth will review highlights from Session 6.
⏱ **Time:**	10 minutes
✂ **Materials:**	None

Procedure

1 After the opening ritual, sit down with the youth and catch up on any business. Ask if anyone has new field assignments to share.

2 Answer any questions from the Question Box.

3 Review Session 6 by asking the following questions:

- What are 2 examples of barrier methods of birth control?

- What kind of lubrication should you use with a condom?

- What is the best type of contraception to avoid HIV and other STD?

- What are several ways you can be close to someone without having sexual intercourse?

2.

Goal Setting: My Future

Source: Planned Parenthood of Maryland's STARS (Students Talking About Responsible Sexuality).

☺	**Objective:**	Youth will identify long-term goals for themselves and learn how to avoid possible obstacles to achieving these goals.
🕐	**Time:**	20 minutes
✂	**Materials:**	8-1/2" x 11" paper, 3 sheets for each participant
		Markers
		Adjustments to the Future cards (See page 160.)

Procedure

1 Discuss the concept of goal setting. Goal setting is defined as deciding what you want to do and the time frame in which you want to accomplish it. Tell the group that this activity is designed to help them establish some long-term goals. Define long-term goals as "goals that cannot be accomplished in a short period of time, like a few days or weeks," and ask for several examples from the group.

2 Give each youth 3 pieces of paper and a marker. Ask them to draw 1 picture on each sheet to represent an accomplishment they want to achieve between now and age 25. Give them some examples such as owning a house, going to college, traveling all over the world, writing a book or having a good job. Group leaders should complete this activity too (choose goals for the next 10 years).

3 Invite each person to show his or her goals to the group.

4 Mention that everyone needs to be prepared for the unexpected in the future, because things do not always proceed according to plans. Give each participant an **Adjustments to the Future** card. Remind them that this is just a game.

5 The group leader should go first. (*Note:* Make sure you have a card with a negative impact, such as selling drugs, testing positive for HIV, or getting fired for testing positive for drugs.) Discuss how this will make it very difficult to accomplish some of your goals.

6 Go around to each participant and discuss how their "adjustment to the future" would affect their ability to accomplish their goals. Ask:

- Is there a way you can make sure this adjustment happens? (for positive adjustments)

- Is there a way you can make sure it doesn't happen? (for negative adjustments)

- If negative things DO happen, how can you continue to work toward your goals?

7 Lead a discussion about goal setting, using some or all of the following questions:

- What things do people consider when setting goals for the future?

- Do youth usually set goals that are based on reality or fantasy?

- How flexible are most people when things don't go as planned?

- At what age are most teens planning to get their first job? Get married? Start a family?

- Do youth think about how their present behavior might influence their future goals? Do kids feel vulnerable or invulnerable?

- (When applicable) How might someone avoid negative adjustments?

- (When applicable) How might someone ensure that positive adjustments happen?

- What are some things that could happen that you may not be able to control?

(*Note:* It is important for youth to know what they can control, *and* how to deal with things beyond their control, such as a relative's death or illness, or being laid off from a job.)

8 Summarize by stating that there are some adjustments that you can plan for and some that you can not. They have been learning skills that will help them plan so they can reach their goals. Youth need to practice good sexual health and prevent unplanned pregnancy, HIV and other STD to ensure that they achieve their goals.

As they saw in the lesson, things don't always go as planned, so they need to know how to make the best of a situation even though their plans have changed. Remind them they can ask for help from parents or other adults when they run into barriers.

Card Master

Adjustments to the Future

Copy and cut apart the cards. Make enough to have 1 card for each participant.

1.

You graduated from high school.

6.

You got a scholarship for college.

2.

You dropped out of high school.

7.

You tested positive for HIV.

3.

You were arrested for selling drugs.

8.

You had a baby your senior year in high school.

4.

You never got married.

9.

You were laid off from your job.

5.

You got offered a manager position at McDonald's while in high school.

10.

You were fired from your job because you tested positive for drugs.

3. Images of Sex

☺ **Objective:** Youth will explore their positive and negative ideas and feelings about sex.

Youth will define sexual health for themselves.

🕐 **Time:** 30 minutes

✂ **Materials:** Cards, crayons, newsprint, markers, tape and scissors

---

Procedure

1 Introduce the activity by stating that today they will talk about images of sex. Explain that sex is something relevant to all of us. As youth we have seen our bodies changing as we grow and, for most of us, part of becoming an adult is the expectation of having children. When we are ready for sex, it should be enjoyable, fun and rewarding for both people.

Note that NONE of us would have been born if it wasn't for sex! But at the same time, almost all of us at some time in our lives have questions or difficulties related to sex, which we may find painful or embarrassing, but with which we would like some help. Acknowledge that help is often hard to find.

Explain that this activity is a way to help us share with one another our own understanding of the good things and the difficult things about sex in our own lives. Because people often find it difficult to talk about sex and sexual health, youth are going to draw about it instead.

Notes for Group Leaders: If you are doing this with youth who are not yet sexually active, you could ask them instead to draw hopes and fears that they have about sex.

---

2 Ask youth to divide into small groups of 3 or 4. Give each group at least 10 small index cards and a small pack of crayons. Explain that you would like them to draw 1 aspect of sex or something they feel connects in some way to sex on each card. They can use as many cards as they would like.

Explain that the aspect can be good or bad, funny, happy or sad, and that the images do not have to be skillfully drawn. As long as their small group understands the meaning of what has been drawn, that is good enough.

3 Give each small group up to 10 minutes to draw on as many cards as they like.

4 While the small groups are busy, lay 4 pieces of newsprint, long end to long end, on the ground and anchor them with tape. Label one end "Good" and the other end "Bad."

5 Call youth back into the big circle, asking them to bring their cards with them.

6 Ask youth to sort through their group's cards and place them near the good end or near the bad end of the newsprint, depending on how they feel about the image they have drawn. If they feel that topics on certain cards are similar or are in some way connected, they should place these cards close to each other.

7 Once all the cards are placed somewhere along the continuum, ask youth to move along the 4 sheets together, starting at the Good end. Each card should be viewed by the entire group. The group who drew the card should describe what they have drawn, so that everyone understands what their picture means. Encourage youth to discuss the subject of each card, so that you and they together have a chance to share and learn about the issues raised.

8 Summarize that sexual health can be defined as "sexual expression that is pleasurable for both people, and free from infection, unwanted pregnancy and abuse." Since each group is likely to have its own particular issues to include in this definition, work with youth to expand the definition.

Notes for Group Leaders: This can be a valuable opportunity for youth and you to learn from one another what is known about sexual health in this peer group. If youth prefer not to talk about themselves, you can encourage them to talk about issues they have heard about from others. In this way, youth often manage to talk about themselves, but in a way which feels less personal for them.

This activity enables youth to share their worries with one other, and you can learn about problems they may have that are not being addressed. It also gives you an opportunity to learn what priority—if any—these youth give to the prevention of HIV and other STD, compared to other sexual health matters.

4.

Roleplay: Saying NO or Asking to Use a Condom

☺ **Objective:**   Youth will practice communication skills to carry out their decisions.

🕐 **Time:**   20 minutes

✂ **Materials:**   Newsprint

Props for the roleplay (e.g., hats or scarves)

Procedure

1 Review the assertive communication style discussed in Session 5. Write the following guidelines on newsprint:

- Be clear about what you want.

- Keep your voice strong but not too loud.

- Make eye contact with the other person.

- Stand up straight.

- Be confident and respect your feelings.

- Respect the other person.

2 Explain that roleplaying allows youth to take on the role of another person. They can practice feeling, talking and acting like someone else. It also helps them learn new options for dealing with a problem and allows them to practice new skills.

3 Have youth pair up and each prepare a roleplay. Have 1 youth be Chantel or Tavon and the other be the boyfriend or girlfriend. Have them roleplay telling a partner they don't want to have sex or asking the partner to use a condom.

If they get stuck, instruct them to look at the guidelines on newsprint for help. If you have time, have volunteers do their roleplay in front of the group.

4 Lead a discussion about the roleplay using the following questions:

- Was the roleplay realistic? Why or why not?

- What kind of communication did you see?

- How do the guidelines help?

- *For actors:* How did you feel in your roles?

- *For audience:* Do you want to change or add anything to the way the actors communicated?

- What other options did roleplayers come up with to solve the problem?

5. Wrap-Up and Closing Ritual

☺ **Objective:**	Youth will provide feedback on Session 7 and summarize what they have learned.
◷ **Time:**	5 minutes
✄ **Materials:**	Field Assignment worksheets

Procedure

1 Have the group sit in a circle. Perform the chosen closing ritual.

2 Gather feedback about the day's session by asking the following questions:

- What did they like?

- What didn't they like?

- What did they learn?

- What would they like to learn more about at another session?

3 Remind youth of the next meeting time and place. State that this will be the last session and encourage them all to come. Tell them to remind each other. Offer to give them a call the night before the meeting. Remind them that they can still do field assignments. Have worksheets available for them.

4 Provide a way for youth to contact you if they need to and remind them that they can use the Question Box.

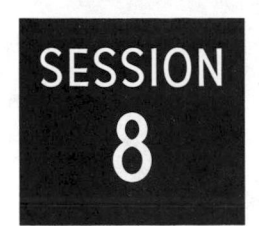

SESSION 8

Review and Community Project

Purpose   Youth will build self-efficacy about HIV/STD prevention.

Session Overview
(90 minutes)

1 Opening Ritual and Review (10 minutes)

2 The Knowledge Feud (20 minutes)

3 Pat on the Back (20 minutes)

4 Community Projects Discussion (30 minutes)

5 Wrap-Up and Closing Ritual (10 minutes)

Preparation

Pre-Session Activities

❑ Read over and become familiar with Session 8 activities.

❑ Prepare snacks.

❑ Staple a 2 ft. loop of yarn to the top of each paper plate

❑ Copy **Activity Planning Sheet** for each participant. (See pages 180–181.)

Materials

❑ snacks

❑ SODA Model and Groundrules charts

❑ newsprint

❑ markers

❑ clock

❑ paper plates to write on

❑ pens or pencils

❑ masking tape

❑ **Activity Planning Sheet,** 1 for each participant

I.

Opening Ritual and Review

☺ **Objective:**	Youth will review highlights from Session 7.
🕐 **Time:**	10 minutes
✂ **Materials:**	None

Procedure

1 After the opening ritual, sit down with youth and catch up on any business. Ask if anyone has new field assignments to share.

2 Answer any questions from the Question Box.

3 Review Session 7 by asking the following questions:

- How would you define *sexual health*?

- What is a long-term goal?

- What are some elements of effective communication?

2.

The Knowledge Feud

Source: Planned Parenthood of Maryland's STARS (Students Talking About Responsible Sexuality).

☺ **Objective:**   Youth review knowledge of HIV/STD prevention and increase their belief in their ability to protect themselves from infection.

🕐 **Time:**   20 minutes

✂ **Materials:**   Clock

Game Questions, for group leader (See pages 172–174.)

Procedure

1   Divide the group into 2 teams. Explain that they will play a game to review some of the things they have learned in the *Focus on Kids* program.

2   Explain the rules for the "game":

- The group leader will read a question to each team. The team picked to go first (decided by flipping a coin) will have 3 seconds to give a correct answer. If they answer correctly, they again have 3 seconds to come up with another correct response.

- This process continues until the first team cannot think of a correct answer or guesses incorrectly. If the first team runs out of time or answers incorrectly, the question passes to the second team.

- The second team then has the opportunity to finish answering the question.

- If a team gets all the correct responses to a question, they have earned 1 point.

- Once a team has earned a point, the next question goes to the other team.

- This process continues until all the questions are answered.

- The group leader will write up the points on newsprint as they are earned. The team with the most points wins!

3 Starting with the team that won the coin toss, ask one of the **Game Questions.** Continue with the game until all questions have been answered. (*Note:* You can add other questions if desired.)

4 Summarize by saying that youth have learned a lot from the *Focus on Kids* program and they need to make sure they use this knowledge to lead healthy lives and achieve their goals.

Game Questions

- What are 7 steps in using a condom properly?

    1. Buy or get latex condoms. (Be sure they are latex, not lambskin, because the pores of lambskin condoms are larger and therefore it is possible for the HIV virus to get through the pores.)

    2. Check the expiration date on the back of the condom package.

    3. Discuss safer sex with your partner before you are aroused.

    4. Place the condom on the man's erect penis.

    5. Squeeze the air out of the tip of the condom. Make sure there is a space between the end of the penis and the condom to collect the semen.

    6. Unroll the condom over the penis all the way to the base of the penis. Continue to hold on to the tip while you roll the condom down.

    7. After intercourse, hold on to the rim of the condom while removing the penis (so the condom does not stay inside the partner).

    8. Throw condom away properly. (Wrap in toilet paper and throw away in a trash can. Do not flush it down the toilet.)

- What are 5 different activities we did in the program?

- What are 3 modes of transmission for HIV?

    – Exchange of body fluids (semen, vaginal fluids, blood, breastmilk), sharing needles (exchange of blood), from pregnant mother to child.

- What are 5 things that occur during puberty for boys?

    – Testicles gradually grow larger and fuller

    – Penis gradually grows larger and longer

    – Body sweats more

    – Skin and hair become more oily

    – Soft, darker hair grows around the base of the penis and later becomes curly, thick and coarse

Game Questions (continued)

- Hair grows under the arms

- Hair grows on the face, first the mustache then the beard and sideburns

- Hair may grow on chest

- The voice cracks and then becomes deeper

- Sperm begin to be produced

- Ejaculations—including wet dreams—begin to occur

- **What are 5 things that occur during puberty for girls?**

    - Body sweats more

    - Skin and hair become more oily

    - Body has sudden growth spurt

    - Soft, darker hair grows around the vulva and later becomes curly, thick and coarse

    - Hair grows under the arms

    - Breasts and nipples gradually grow larger and fuller

    - Nipples may become a darker color

    - Menstrual periods begin

- **What are 4 feelings that can be communicated nonverbally and verbally?**

    - Any feelings—sadness, disgust, happiness, anger, fear, silliness, etc.

- **What are the 4 parts of the SODA Decision-Making Model?**

    - Step 1: **S**top—**Stop and state the problem.**

    - Step 2: **O**ptions—**Consider the options** or choices and the consequences of those choices.

    - Step 3: **D**ecide—**Decide and choose the best solution** from the options.

    - Step 4: **A**ction—**Act on your decision.**

Game Questions (continued)

- Demonstrate 5 elements of assertive behavior.

    – Content: specific, direct, problem-oriented, suggest solutions

    – Voice: clear, moderate in tone

    – Facial expression: eye contact

    – Posture: erect, comfortable

    – Your feelings: confident, self-respecting, comfortable

    – The other's feelings: respected

    – Goal of the behavior: a change in the situation

- What are 3 types of barrier methods?

    – Male condom, female condom, diaphragm and spermicide

- What are 5 advantages of barrier methods?

    – Don't need a prescription.

    – Can purchase from drugstore (or get for free at clinic).

    – Protect against pregnancy.

    – Condoms (male and female) protect against HIV and STD.

    – No major side effects.

- Name 8 places where you can get information.

    – Phone books, teachers, parents, other adults, hotlines, libraries, clinics, school, books, doctors and nurses, etc.

3.

Pat on the Back

Source: Planned Parenthood of Maryland's STARS (Students Talking About Responsible Sexuality).

☺ **Objective:** Youth will give compliments to each other.

🕐 **Time:** 20 minutes

✂ **Materials:** Paper plates, with a 2 ft loop of yarn stapled to the top so the plate can be worn around the neck with the plate on the person's back

Pens or pencils

Procedure

1 Have youth stand in a circle. Give each person a paper plate. Have them put the yarn around their necks with the plate hanging on their backs.

2 Explain the activity:

- Starting with the person in front of you, write down 1 positive thing you have learned about or from that person.

- You do not have to sign your name to the comment, but it must be positive and supportive.

3 Have youth move around and try to "pat" everyone's back by writing 1 positive thing about that person on his or her plate. Make sure that all plates are written on by the majority of the group members.

4 Return to the original circle and ask youth to look at their plates. Give them a minute to read their plates privately.

5 Starting with the group leader, have each person share 1 compliment that was written on his or her plate.

6 Summarize by saying that it is obvious they all have a lot of good characteristics. Remind youth that compliments enhance how we think about ourselves, and that when we feel good about ourselves we make decisions that help us protect ourselves and reach our goals. Tell them they should all feel very good about themselves and make good decisions in the future.

4. Community Projects Discussion

Source: Adapted from Center for Population Options' Guide to Implementing TAP (Teens for AIDS Prevention Peer Education Program).

☺ **Objective:** Youth increase their self-efficacy about HIV/STD prevention by sharing their knowledge and attitudes with others in their community.

🕐 **Time:** 30 minutes

✂ **Materials:** Paper and pencils for all group members

List of **Possible Community Projects,** for group leader (See page 179.)

Activity Planning Sheet worksheet

Procedure

1 Give each youth a piece of paper and ask them to write down their skills and interests (e.g. to rap, to act, to write, to draw, to play sports, to teach, to sing, etc.) Ask youth to write their names on the paper.

Collect the papers. Without naming names, review the general strengths, skills and interests of the individuals in the group. Tell youth to keep these things in mind when choosing a project.

2 Share the examples of **Possible Community Projects.** The projects do not need to be related to HIV. Youth can choose from any of the things their group has discussed during the program.

If this is not a group that will be able to meet again, they should choose something that can be completed in this last session. If the group is a group that *will* continue to meet, they could choose something more long term. One option is to put together a performance for the audience at the graduation ceremony.

3 Once youth have determined what they are going to do have them fill out an **Activity Planning Sheet** as a group. Younger youth may need help filling out the sheet.

Notes for Group Leaders: If the project is going to have to be completed in 1 session, the group leaders should gather a variety of materials ahead of time so that the project can be done during this time.

If this is a group that will continue to meet, the group leaders will need to review the **Activity Planning Sheets** to determine what supplies will need to be purchased and what preparation is necessary (e.g., ask schools about putting up posters, arrange a time with rec club director for assembly, etc.).

Group Leader

Possible Community Projects

Buttons

- Students in Washington, D.C. developed buttons with HIV prevention messages. They gave these buttons to their friends and acquaintances.

  The buttons served as an informal medium for the students to communicate about HIV and AIDS with their friends.

Bulletin Boards

- At another school, a bulletin board located in a busy hallway was covered with the latest HIV articles from newspapers and magazines.

  Posters and HIV prevention messages can be posted on bulletin boards, as well as hotline numbers for additional information. Some of the most commonly asked questions about HIV and AIDS and the answers can also be posted.

Posters

- Youth can design and draw posters incorporating the latest youth language. The posters can be put in schools, rec clubs, community bulletin boards, local record stores, fast-food restaurants, etc.

Assemblies

- Youth can organize an assembly where a guest speaker (possibly a person with HIV, someone who was a teen parent, a recovered drug user or a ex-drug-dealer) can come speak to a group about his or her personal experiences.

- Youth speakouts can be held, in which youth discuss why they feel it is important for their age group to think about HIV and avoid risk behaviors.

- Youth can also organize assemblies where videos the youth enjoyed are shown and discussed.

- Assemblies can also incorporate theater skits, raps or formal presentations by the group.

Writing

- Youth can write articles for school, community or city newspapers (including a *Focus on Kids* newsletter).

- Youth can organize an essay contest on one of the subjects they have explored during their training.

Videos

- Youth can put skits or vignettes on video for others to view.

Activity Planning Sheet

Group members' names: _____

_____

The goal of the activity is: _____

_____

Describe the activity: _____

_____

_____

What is/are the main message(s) that will be conveyed?_____

_____

_____

What skills will the people you are teaching learn? _____

_____

_____

How many people will be reached? _____

When will the activity occur (date)?_____

Where will the activity occur?_____

What materials will you need? _____

_____

(continued)

Worksheet

(Activity Planning Sheet, continued)

Tasks that need to be done:	By whom?	By when?
_____	_____	_____
_____	_____	_____
_____	_____	_____
_____	_____	_____
_____	_____	_____

Estimated budget: _____

_____

_____

_____

5.

Wrap-Up and Closing Ritual

☺ **Objective:** Youth will provide feedback on the program and summarize what they have learned.

🕐 **Time:** 10 minutes

✂ **Materials:** None

Procedure

1 Have the group sit in a circle. Perform the closing ritual.

2 Gather feedback about the day's session and the entire program by asking the following questions:

- What did they like?

- What didn't they like?

- What did they learn?

- What did they think of the Focus on Kids program?

- Are there other things they would include in the program?

3 If you've planned a graduation ceremony (see page 9), remind youth of the graduation date. Tell them to remind each other.

Resource Section

Sample Parent Letter

Date: _____

Dear Parent,

The (name of site) is offering an HIV-prevention program to youth 9–15 years of age. In the program, youth will learn how to protect themselves from HIV infection. This will be done by learning knowledge and skills such as decision making, abstaining from sex, condom use, negotiation and communication. Youth will learn these skills by playing games, watching videos and having group discussions.

The program will be held every _____ day at _____ (time) for 8 weeks. The youth should enjoy and have fun with the program.

If you would like your child to participate in this program please sign the attached permission slip and send it back to the Center. If you have any questions about the program now or any time in the future, please call me at _____.

Sincerely,

Name _____

Title _____

Name of Center _____

Sample Parent Permission Slip

I agree to let my child participate in the *Focus on Kids* program being done by _____(name of site). I understand that if my child participates in the program, she/he will be taught information on decision making, abstinence, condom use, communication skills and learn specific information about HIV and how to avoid it.

I understand that all discussions that my child will have with the group leaders of this project will be confidential and will not be reported to me or anyone else.

I agree to let my child participate in this program. I understand that she/he is free to stop at any time.

Youth's name _____

Age _____

Parent or Guardian's signature _____

Date _____

Address_____

Phone _____

Group leader's signature _____

Date _____

Parent Information Session Outline

Purpose
To overview the objectives and approaches of the *Focus on Kids* program.

To answer parents' questions and concerns about the program.

Sample Agenda

- **Introduction Activity—Flying Objects** (10 minutes) (See Session 1, Activity 1A.)

- *Focus on Kids* **Program Overview** (20 minutes)

- **Model Sample Program Activities** (45 minutes)

  - Overview of SODA Decision-Making Model (Session 1)

  - How Risky Is It? (Session 2)

  - Communication Roleplay (Session 5)

- **Question-and-Answer Period** (15 minutes)

Optional All-Day Retreat for Session 6

Purpose
The all-day retreat includes the learning activities from Session 6 as well as a variety of recreational activities. The retreat offers an opportunity for boys' and girls' groups to work together as well as hear a presentation by an outside speaker.

Sample Agenda

(10:00-10:15) Introduction Game and Opening Ritual

(10:15-10:20) Review of Session 5

(10:20-10:40) Ways to Show You Care

(10:40-10:55) HIV Transmission Game

(10:55-12:00) Recreational Activities (e.g., relays, tug-of-war, hikes, scavenger hunt, etc.)

(12:00-12:45) Lunch

(12:45-1:45) Outside Speaker

(1:45-2:30) Contraception Lesson

(2:30-3:15) Recreational Activities

(3:15-3:30) Wrap-Up and Closing Ritual

Notes for Group Leaders: To make the retreat successful, group leaders will need to prepare for Session 6 (See pages 133–153.) as well as for the retreat. Preparation for the retreat is described on the following page.

Pre-Session Activities

❏ Find a park or camp to use for the retreat. Be sure it has some sheltered areas in case of bad weather.

❏ Reserve the park for a date that works for the groups involved.

❏ Schedule appropriate transportation.

❏ Send out permission slips with youth at least 2 weeks prior to the retreat. Make sure permission slips cover legal considerations that your organization and the park require. It is also important to make sure you have health insurance information for youth and know where the closest hospital is to the park.

❏ Arrange for lunch.

❏ Decide on the structured recreational activities: relays, tug-of-war, hikes, scavenger hunts, etc.

Materials

❏ first-aid kit

❏ plenty of liquids

❏ lunches

❏ permission slips for all youth

❏ recreational activity supplies

Tips on Soliciting Donations

- **Carry "professional begging" letters** and information about the program with you wherever you go (e.g., movies, restaurants, grocery stores, malls, etc.). It never hurts to ask for a donation.

- **Get started early.** It may take a long time for a donation to be approved and go through the chain of command, often as long as a month. Also, many organizations have limits on how much they donate each year and once they've fulfilled their quotas they stop giving donations.

- **Use the yellow pages** to get ideas. Call an agency or business and ask for the manager. If he or she is not able to help, ask for the corporate headquarters.

- **Local fast food chains,** such as McDonald's, are almost always good for orange drink, cups, napkins and cookies.

Sample Donations Letter

Organization name _____

Organization address_____

Date _____

To whom it may concern,

The Youth Development Center at _____(name, site)
offers youth in the community cultural, recreational, tutoring and
health education activities. The center provides after-school, evening
and weekend programs designed to address many of the challenges
facing youth in our community, including substance abuse,
involvement in crime and violence, truancy and pregnancy. The
program goals are to keep our youth off the streets and involved in
positive activities.

The Center has established an HIV-prevention program called *Focus
on Kids*. Youth meet weekly for 8 weeks to focus on decision making;
goal setting; communication skills; and factual information about
avoiding HIV infection, teen pregnancy and drug use. The goal of the
program is to aid youth to make healthy decisions about their lives.

It is our hope that your company might be able to provide products
that could be used as incentives for youth who successfully
participate in this program. Food items for snacks or small gift items
would be extremely helpful in ensuring that youth take part in this
positive program.

If you have any questions, please do not hesitate to contact me at
_____. Thank you in advance for your cooperation.

Sincerely yours,

Name _____

Title _____

Name of Center _____

Background Information on Adolescent Development

Adolescence is a time of change and transitions. Many things are happening at the same time, which may be confusing both to adolescents and the adults around them

Biological

Adolescents go through many important transitions as their hormones begin to signal changes in their development. Hormonal changes trigger the development of secondary sex characteristics (changes in voice, hair growth, etc.). Hormones also are related to emotional changes, characterized by rapid mood swings or what may appear to be overly emotional reactions. These reactions may be confusing to teens themselves as well as to those around them.

Physical

Individual adolescents experience growth spurts at different times. While one 12-year-old boy may suddenly grow tall and muscular, his friend of the same age may still be short and slight in build. One girl may have begun her menstrual cycle and have developed a mature-looking body while her same-age friend may still look more like a little girl.

These changes become important to a youth's self-image, and to her or his status among peers. Adults need to be sensitive to these issues, since adolescents are sensitive to them and may react to them quite strongly.

Adults also need to keep in mind that physical growth and changes in the way youth think do not always keep pace with each other. It may be necessary to remind ourselves that the tall and muscular boy is not necessarily more mature or advanced cognitively and emotionally than his small friend. Our expectations of what is age-appropriate behavior should not be guided by a youth's physical appearance.

Psychological

Cognitive Skills

As youth go from preadolescence into adolescence, their ability to think about situations and concepts develops considerably. Preadolescents are more likely to think about things concretely, and need many examples before they can grasp the meaning of a concept. As adolescents mature, they gain the ability to think more abstractly. They begin to enjoy thinking and talking more about abstract concepts, and to consider possibilities and hypothetical situations.

This becomes an exciting time for them as they become more aware of their own mental abilities and imagination. If you can capture that imagination, it will make your lessons that much more interesting to them.

Identity

During the course of development, adolescents may fall on different points along this continuum, as they try to negotiate their way into becoming autonomous young adults. However, this is not a smooth process, and the same adolescent may be at either extreme within a matter of moments.

Dependence   Autonomy

As adults, it is our task to assist them in negotiating this transition, while recognizing that they may sometimes need to take a few steps back before taking a full stride forward.

Primarily because of this struggle for independence and autonomy, at times you may be challenged by youths' behaviors. Keep in mind that behaviors are one method of communication. If an adolescent misbehaves, your first question to yourself should be, "What is this adolescent trying to tell me?" You must also decide how to handle misbehavior and respond to the youth, while ensuring that the group as a whole continues to move smoothly. The Tips on Managing Behavior section may give you some ideas.

Interpersonal

Relationship with Parents

Issues of power and control can be difficult for adolescents and may be a source of conflict with parents. Adolescents seem to develop best in situations where there are moderate levels of control (neither total freedom nor excessive control), with adults who communicate an atmosphere of emotional support and caring.

Relationships with Peers

Relationships with peers are extremely important during adolescence as part of identity formation. Adolescents often look to friends for feedback, for example about their looks, behaviors and choices. Saving face is extremely important, especially since adolescents are easily embarrassed. It is important to recognize that one reason for misbehavior may be the need to save face or to maintain a favorable perception in friends' eyes.

PROGRAMS
that
WORK✓

Focus on Kids
HIV Awareness
Curriculum Fact Sheet

Target Audience

Youth, ages 9–15, from 9 recreation centers in urban, low-income neighborhoods of Baltimore, Maryland. All youth were African American.

Length

8 sessions; 7 1-1/2 hours and 1 all-day outing

Behavioral Findings

Six months after the program, condom use was significantly higher among *Focus on Kids* participants (especially boys) than for those in the control group.

Objectives

At the completion of this program, participants will be able to:

- State correct information about HIV, AIDS and other STD including modes of transmission and prevention.

- State their own personal values and understand how these relate to pressures to engage in sexual risk behaviors.

- Be skilled in decision making, communicating and negotiating with other youth regarding sexual topics and drug topics, and be able to use a condom correctly.

Materials

A curriculum guide that includes an Implementation section with instructions for group leaders, lesson plans, activity guides, handouts for duplication, consent forms, and other materials relevant to program implementation and a 30-minute video that provides information about sex and puberty.

Special Features

- The program was delivered to single-gender groups of youth who were already friends. Where possible, use of naturally occurring friendship groups may be a useful adjunct to the program. Although the groups were single gender for the 7 short sessions, the groups were combined for the day-long outing.

- An ongoing, weekly story about a fictional family is used to contextualize decision making and risk.

- In one session, youth develop community projects to practice working with others.

Theories

Focus on Kids is based on Protection Motivation Theory, a social cognitive theory which emphasizes the balance between pressures to engage in the risk behavior (social and personal rewards), risks involved (severity of and personal vulnerability to the undesired outcome), and considerations of the alternatives (effectiveness of the alternative in avoiding the undesirable outcome, ability of the youth to employ the alternative behavior and costs associated with employing the alternative). (Rogers, R. W. 1983. Cognitive and physiological processes in fear appraisals and attitude change: A revised theory of protection motivation. In *Social Psychology*, ed. T. Cacioppi and R. E. Petty, 153-176. New York: Guilford Press.)

Recommended Training

A 2-day training is recommended for group leaders. Trainings include: (a) discussions of implementation issues; (b) modeling of program content and teaching strategies; and (c) practice for effective implementation.

To Order Materials or Arrange for Training

Contact the publisher, ETR Associates, 1-800-321-4407 for program materials. Contact Jennifer Galbraith at the University of Maryland, 1-410-706-4267, to arrange training. Many states may be able to provide information and training on this curriculum. To find out if your state has developed that capacity, call the HIV prevention coordinator at your state department of education.

PROGRAMS
that
WORK✓

Focus on Kids
HIV Awareness
Evaluation Fact Sheet

Intervention

In the spring of 1993, youth ages 9 to 15 were recruited from 9 recreation centers in urban, low-income neighborhoods in Baltimore, Maryland, to attend 8 weekly sessions of an HIV risk reduction intervention. Grounded in a social cognitive theory (Protection Motivation Theory) and developed to be culturally appropriate for the target audience, the intervention provided facts about HIV and AIDS, and emphasized skills development with regard to communication, decision making and condom use. The youth formed intervention groups consisting of 2-10 same-gender friends who were within 3 years of age of each other. In addition to condom use, abstinence and avoidance of substance use and drug trafficking were emphasized in the curriculum.

Research Design

The 76 naturally formed peer groups consisting of 383 youth ages 9-15 were randomly assigned to receive the *Focus on Kids* intervention (n=206) or a control condition (n=177). The control condition consisted of 8 sessions that provided facts about HIV and AIDS prevention, but did not emphasize skills development with regard to negotiation, communication or condom use and was not delivered to the naturally occurring groups of friends.

Participants completed questionnaires via a "talking" Macintosh computer at baseline and 6 months after the intervention. Measures assessed actual risk behaviors, perceptions of risk behaviors and intentions.

Behavioral Findings

At baseline, condom-use rates did not differ significantly. At the 6-month follow-up, rates were significantly higher among intervention than control youth (85% vs 61%, P<.05). The intervention was especially strong among boys (85% vs 57%, P<.05) and among teens ages 13-15 (95% vs 60%, p<.01).

Other Significant Findings

Youth did not differ in their intentions to use condoms at baseline, but in the post-intervention period, intervention youth were significantly more likely than control youth to intend to use a condom. Likewise, in the post-intervention period, intervention youth perceived greater peer use of condoms and increased personal vulnerability to HIV.

B. S. Stanton, X. Li, I. Ricardo, J. Galbraith, S. Feigelman and L. Kaljee. A randomized, controlled effectiveness trial of an AIDS prevention program for low-income African-American youths. *Archives of Pediatrics and Adolescent Medicine* 150:363-372.